Sleep Better

WITH ESSENTIAL OIL

Rebecca Park Totilo

COPYRIGHT

DISCLAIMER

The information contained in this book is intended for educational purposes only and is not meant to substitute for medical care or prescribe treatment for any specific health condition. Please see a qualified healthcare provider for medical treatment. The author and publisher assume no responsibility or liability for any person or group for any loss, damage, or injury resulting from using or misusing any information in this book. No express or implied guarantee is given regarding the effects of using any of the products described herein.

Paperback ISBN: 978-1-7343258-5-0
Electronic ISBN: 978-1-7343258-6-7

A WORD FROM REBECCA

You've changed into your fuzzy pajamas and climbed into a bed with fresh, crisp sheets. You lay your head on a soft pillow and begin to feel your breathing slow down, and your eyes grow heavy. In a few short moments, you drift off into a peaceful sleep. The worries of the day vanish, and your mind and body are at rest for the entire night.

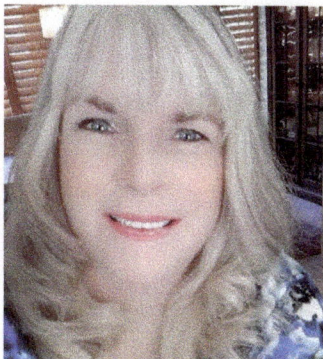

This sounds more like a dream for most people. It can be hard to get optimal sleep in this modern age. Some people have trouble sleeping through the night because of things like a crying baby or a toddler who won't go to bed. For others, a busy work schedule and constant notifications on their phone can be distractions. Even something as small and seemingly insignificant as drinking caffeine during the day or having a lumpy mattress can prevent restful sleep at night. What are we to do when distractions and outside forces steal our sleep?

Fortunately, there is hope for those struggling to get quality, consistent sleep. People worldwide have discovered the potent nature of essential oils to create a restful environment in their homes every night. The aroma of these oils can be combined with other healthy practices before bedtime for an even better experience.

This book will touch on some important aspects of sleeplessness and essential oils. Hopefully, it will answer questions you have on how to use essential oils at bedtime and create a more restful environment for getting the best sleep possible.

Sweet Dreams,

Rebecca Park Totilo

Table of *CONTENTS*

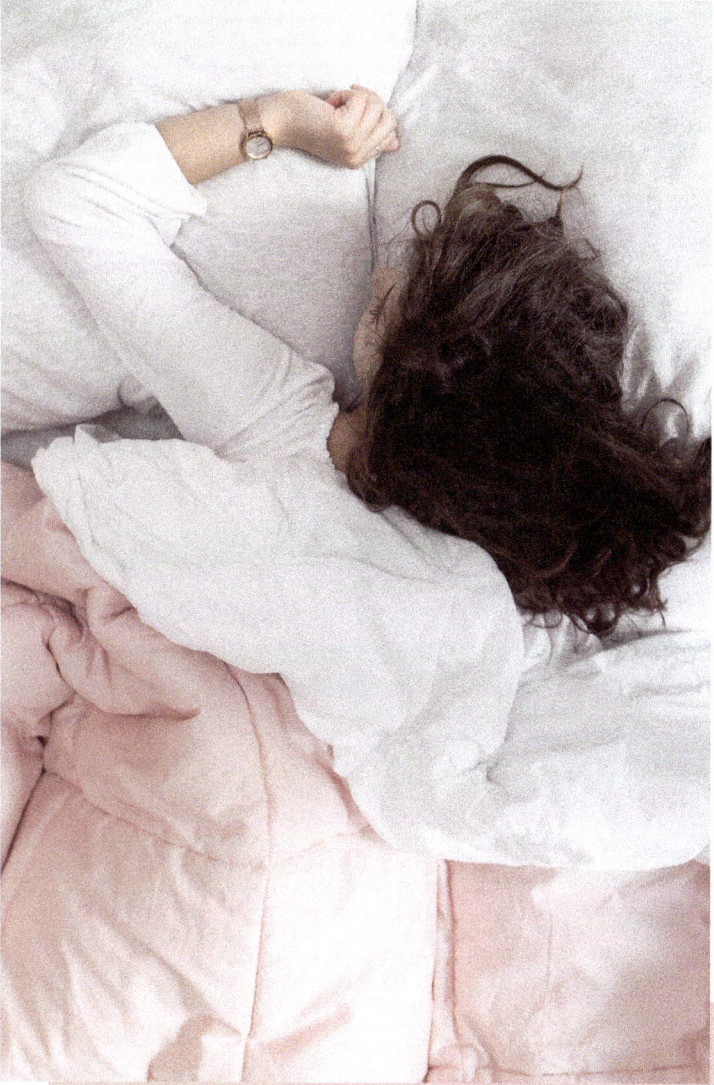

CHAPTER ONE

RISE AND SHINE

How do you feel when you wake up in the morning? Do you feel well-rested? Or do you feel like you were tossing and turning all night? Do you feel invigorated, ready to start your day, or weighed down by poor sleep?

Sleep is one of the most important parts of a healthy life, whether you're an early bird or a night owl. Despite its importance, sleep is one of the most undervalued aspects of modern schedules. We often sacrifice sleep for other things like work, family responsibilities, and even technological distractions.

Indeed, exercise, healthy eating, and finding constructive ways to cope with emotions and stress are all important during the day. However, allowing your mind and body to rest and recover at night is vital. Some may believe the only outcome of poor sleep is feeling tired or sluggish the next day. Yet, sleep deprivation has been linked to various health issues.

Sleeping is more than just getting our beauty rest. When we sleep, our brains and bodies go through significant processes essential for growth, learning and memory, and recovery of bodily systems. Some may think it's a luxury to get quality sleep, but sleep should be viewed not as a luxury but as a necessity—as crucial for survival as food and water.

As we sleep, our brains process the day's information, stimuli, and memories. The brain sorts through important details and memories, clearing out waste and excess information to refresh the mind

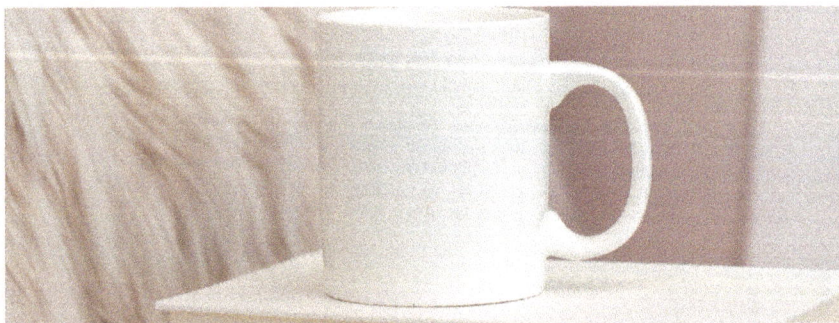

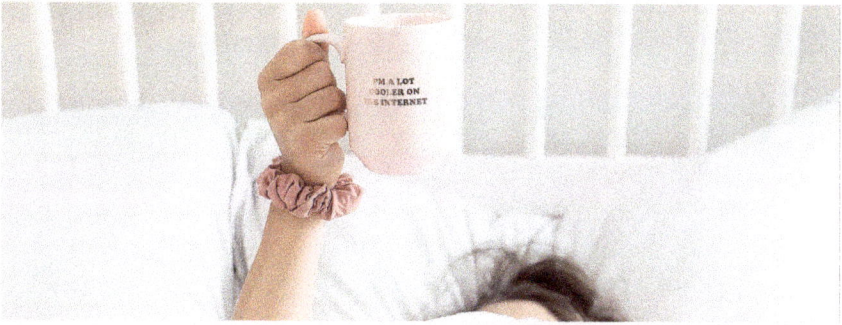

and start fresh in the morning. These processes can be thought of as small but necessary housekeeping items that the brain must complete to keep the rest of the house (the brain) functioning properly. If we miss out on sleep, we aren't giving the brain ample time to refresh or clear away waste, which can ultimately make it more difficult to function properly the next day.

Giving your body a break by getting a good night's sleep will help major systems function as they should. Relaxed, deep sleep allows the body to rest, rejuvenating cells as our muscles relax and we take slow, deep breaths. When we cut these processes short, the body doesn't have time to recuperate, causing problems in the long run.

Nighttime sleep is not just about laying your head down on the pillow and waiting for the morning to start it all over again. It is a complex and constantly changing process. During the night, humans experience several levels of sleep that help the brain and body rest and recover.

Health issues related to insomnia include sleep apnea and restless leg syndrome.

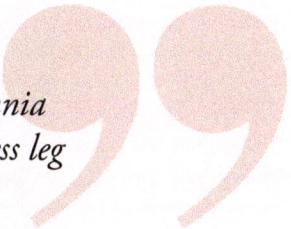

WHAT IS INSOMNIA?

Sleeping difficulties come in many forms. Some people have trouble falling asleep. Others can fall asleep easily but often wake up shortly after. Others may fall asleep and stay asleep, but their sleep is restless and interrupted by bad dreams or physical movement. These sleeping problems usually leave people feeling exhausted the next day. There are various ways to use essential oils to treat these conditions.

Many factors contribute to difficulty falling asleep and staying asleep. Thirty-three percent of Americans report not getting the recommended amount of sleep per night. While some might be tempted to write off their lack of sleep, depriving your body of sleep has a variety of negative impacts on your health. There are several reasons for this, including a higher-stress modern society, electronics, and increased sleep-related problems. Many sleep aids on the market promise to alleviate this issue, but many of these have unwanted side effects.

Insomnia is the inability to sleep despite being tired. Most people have experienced it at one time or another—whether it's a light, fitful sleep that leaves them exhausted or waking up frequently throughout the night or too early.

Researchers debate whether insomnia is always a symptom of another physical or psychological condition or is a primary disorder of its own.

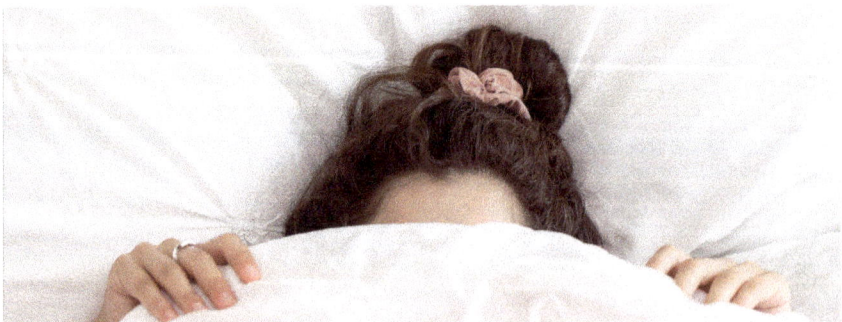

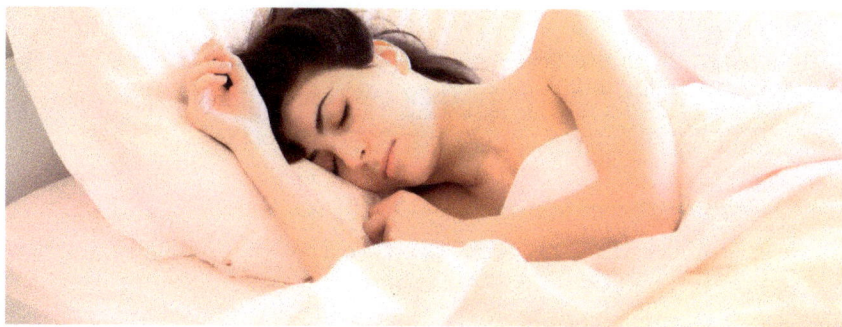

COMMON SYMPTOMS OF INSOMNIA

- Exhausted during the day

- Frequent headaches

- Irritability

- Inability to focus or concentrate

- Wake up groggy and not refreshed

- Sleep better away from home

- Take 30 or 40 minutes to fall asleep

- Repeatedly wake throughout the night

- Wake too early and unable to fall back asleep

- Dependent upon sleep aids

Those with insomnia often complain of being unable to shut off their minds (plagued with unfinished to-do lists, for example). Writers and artistic types claim that they get their best ideas at night while lying in bed trying to sleep.

The worrisome part of insomnia is wanting to sleep but being unable to. The mind recycles the same thoughts repeatedly, making it impossible to rest and then is barely able to function the next day. For some, insomnia lasts only a few nights; for others, it's longer.

Insomnia, usually temporary, is often categorized by how long it lasts, which could be for a few days or last for several weeks. Chronic insomnia is when a person has difficulty falling asleep, maintaining sleep, or has non-restorative rest for several nights or longer. It also can interfere with and impair normal activities due to sleep loss.

Other health issues related to insomnia include sleep apnea and restless leg syndrome. Sleep apnea is a disorder of difficulty breathing during sleep, with persistent, loud snoring and frequent long pauses in breathing during sleep, followed by a gasping for breath.

Restless Leg Syndrome is an unpleasant sensation (creeping, burning, itching, pulling, or tugging) in the legs or feet, occurring primarily in the evening and night.

Circadian Rhythm Disorder is when a person's sleep-wake schedule does not match a natural sleep schedule. People who work the night shift may suffer from this problem. A delayed sleep-phase syndrome is when a circadian clock runs late but reliably. People who experience this condition usually fall asleep late at night or early in the morning but then sleep normally. For older individuals, advanced sleep syndrome produces excessive sleepiness in the wee hours of early morning.

Emotional Issues can also cause sleepless nights of excessive worrying about minor details or sadness due to a lost friend or relative.

CHAPTER TWO

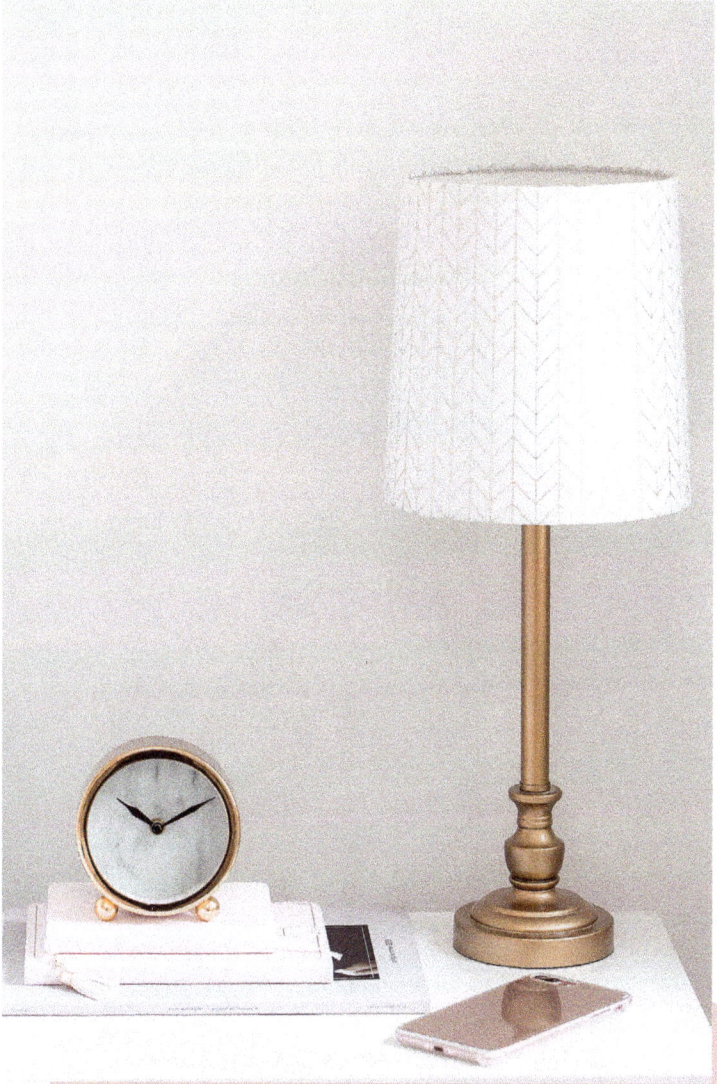

TICK TOCK

Restful sleep is a basic human need for well-being. The daily cycle of life, which includes sleeping and waking, is called a circadian (meaning "about a day") rhythm, commonly referred to as the biological clock. Hundreds of bodily functions follow biological clocks, but sleeping and waking are the most prominent circadian rhythms.

Light signals coming through the eyes reset the circadian cycles each day. The response to light signals in the brain is an important key factor in sleep and maintaining a normal circadian rhythm.

Light signals travel to a tiny cluster of nerves in the hypothalamus in the brain's center, the body's master clock, called the suprachiasmatic nucleus or SCN. This nerve cluster takes its name from its location, just above (supra) the optic chiasm. The optic chiasm is a major junction for nerves transmitting information about light from the eyes.

The approach of dusk each day prompts the SCN to signal the nearby pineal gland (named so because it resembles a pine cone) to produce the hormone melatonin.

Some experts believe melatonin is an important hormone released in the brain critical for the body's time-setting. The longer a person is in darkness, the more prolonged melatonin is secreted. Levels drop after staying in bright light. Research is ongoing to determine if high levels of melatonin cause sleep, regardless of whether it is dark.

The sleep-wake cycles in humans are designed to produce activity

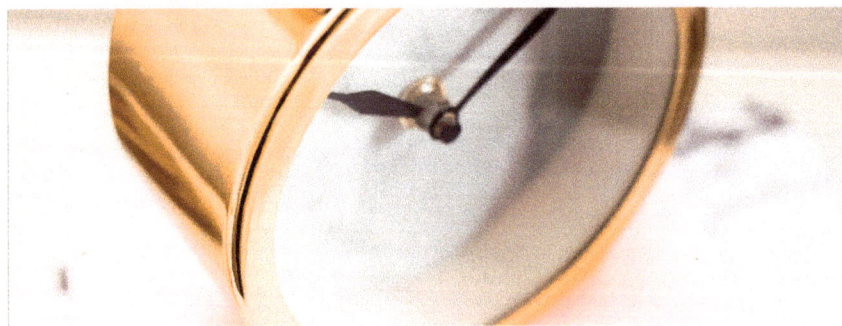

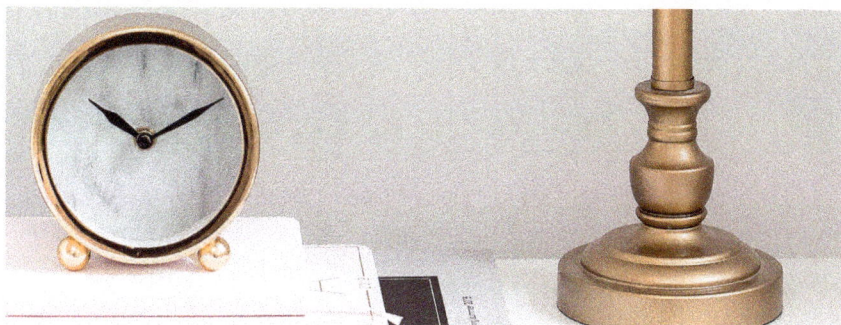

during the day and sleep at night. There is also a natural peak in sleepiness at mid-day, the traditional siesta time. The sleeping and waking cycle is approximately 24 hours. When confined to windowless apartments, with no clocks or other time cues, sleeping and waking as the bodies dictate, humans typically live on slightly longer than a 24-hour cycle.

In sleep studies, subjects spend about one-third of their time asleep, suggesting that most people need about eight hours of sleep each day. Infants may sleep as many as 16 hours a day. However, individual adults differ in how much sleep they need to feel well-rested.

Daily rhythms intermesh with several biological and physical factors that may interfere with or change individual patterns. For example, the firing of nerve cells in the brain may be faster or slower in different individuals. Such differences are fractions of a second, but they can cause variations in a person's sleep type, timing, and duration.

Changes in season or exposure to light and dark often unsettle the sleeping pattern.

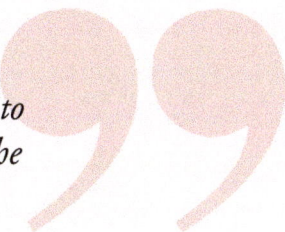

"SLEEP IS MORE THAN JUST GETTING BEAUTY REST."

– ANONYMOUS

SLEEP CYCLES

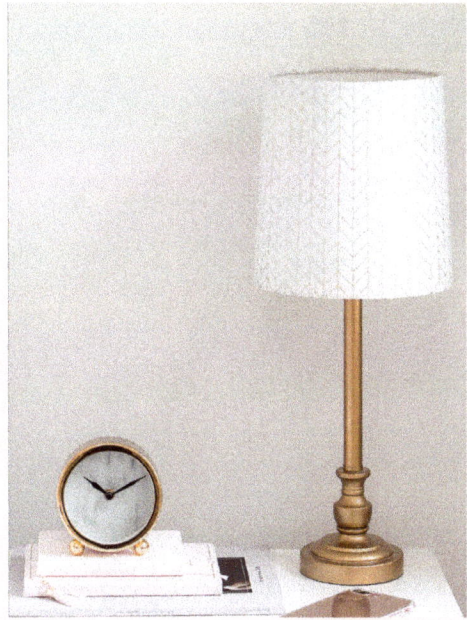

Sleep consists of two distinct states that alternate in cycles and reflect differing brain nerve cell activity levels. One progresses through these stages about five or six times during a typical night's sleep. Non-Rapid Eye Movement Sleep (Non-REM) sleep is also termed quiet sleep. Non-REM is further subdivided into three stages of progression. The sleep process includes three stages of non-rapid eye movement (or NREM) sleep and one stage of rapid eye movement (or REM) sleep. Here is a breakdown of what happens during each of the sleep stages:

SLEEP CONSISTS OF TWO DISTINCT STATES . . .

STAGE 1

LIGHT SLEEP

The first stage is essentially the "dozing off" stage, usually lasting one to five minutes. During this sleep stage, the body hasn't fully relaxed, though the body and brain activities start to slow with periods of brief movements and twitches.

STAGE 2

PROPER SLEEP

The second stage of NREM sleep typically lasts around 20 minutes. During this stage, we usually experience low-frequency brain waves, interrupted by occasional bursts of high-frequency brainwaves. Eye movements stop, body temperature drops, and we enter a period of light sleep.

STAGE 3

DEEP "SLOW-WAVE" OR DELTA SLEEP

The third stage of NREM sleep—termed slow-wave sleep—is a period of deep sleep featuring brainwaves even slower than those in stages one and two. This stage is pivotal for feeling refreshed in the morning. Heart rate and breathing slow significantly, blood pressure decreases, muscles are very relaxed, and waking up is more challenging. This stage typically lasts 20 to 45 minutes.

RAPID EYE

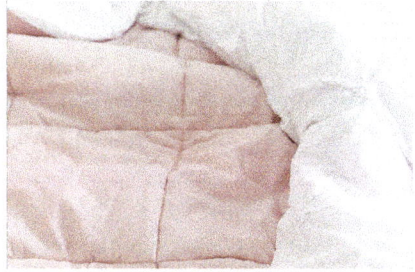

REM sleep occurs approximately 90 minutes after falling asleep and is characterized by intense brain activity, rapid eye movements, faster breathing, and heart rate and blood pressure, similar to waking levels. Most dreaming occurs during this stage, but voluntary muscles like your arms and legs are relaxed. REM sleep is believed to play a role in memory consolidation, learning, and mood regulation. The first REM sleep only lasts around 10 minutes, but it gets progressively longer as you repeat the sleep cycle throughout the night. The final REM sleep can last up to an hour.

With each descending stage, awakening becomes more difficult. It is not known what governs Non-REM sleep in the brain. A balance between certain hormones, particularly growth and stress hormones, may be necessary for deep sleep.

Rapid Eye-Movement Sleep (REM) sleep is termed active sleep, and most vivid dreams occur

MOVEMENT

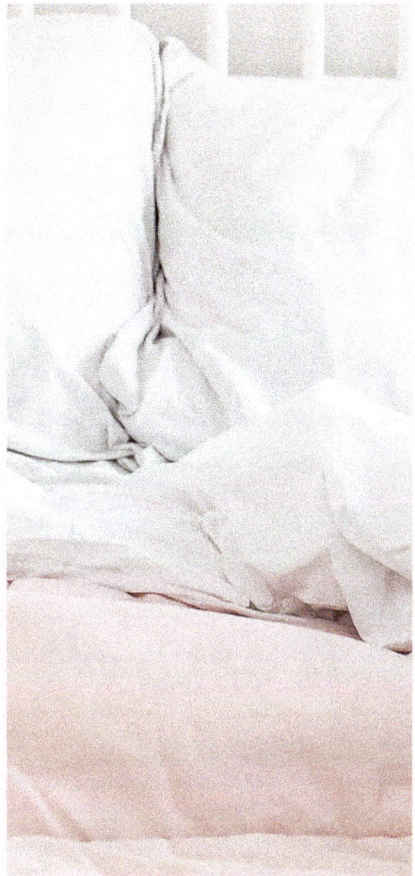

during this stage. REM-sleep brain activity is comparable to waking, but the muscles are virtually paralyzed, possibly preventing people from acting out their dreams.

In fact, except for vital organs like the lungs and heart, the only muscles not paralyzed during REM are the eye muscles. REM sleep may be critical for learning and day-to-day mood regulation. When people are sleep-deprived, their brains must work harder than when they are well-rested.

The cycle between quiet (NREM) and active (REM) sleep follows the same pattern. After about 90 minutes of Non-REM sleep, eyes move rapidly behind closed lids, giving rise to REM sleep. As sleep progresses, the Non-REM/REM cycle repeats. Non-REM sleep becomes progressively lighter with each cycle, and REM sleep becomes longer, lasting from a few minutes early to almost an hour at the end of the sleep episode.

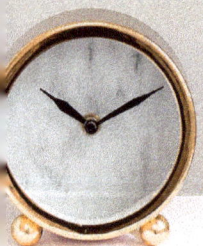

CHAPTER THREE

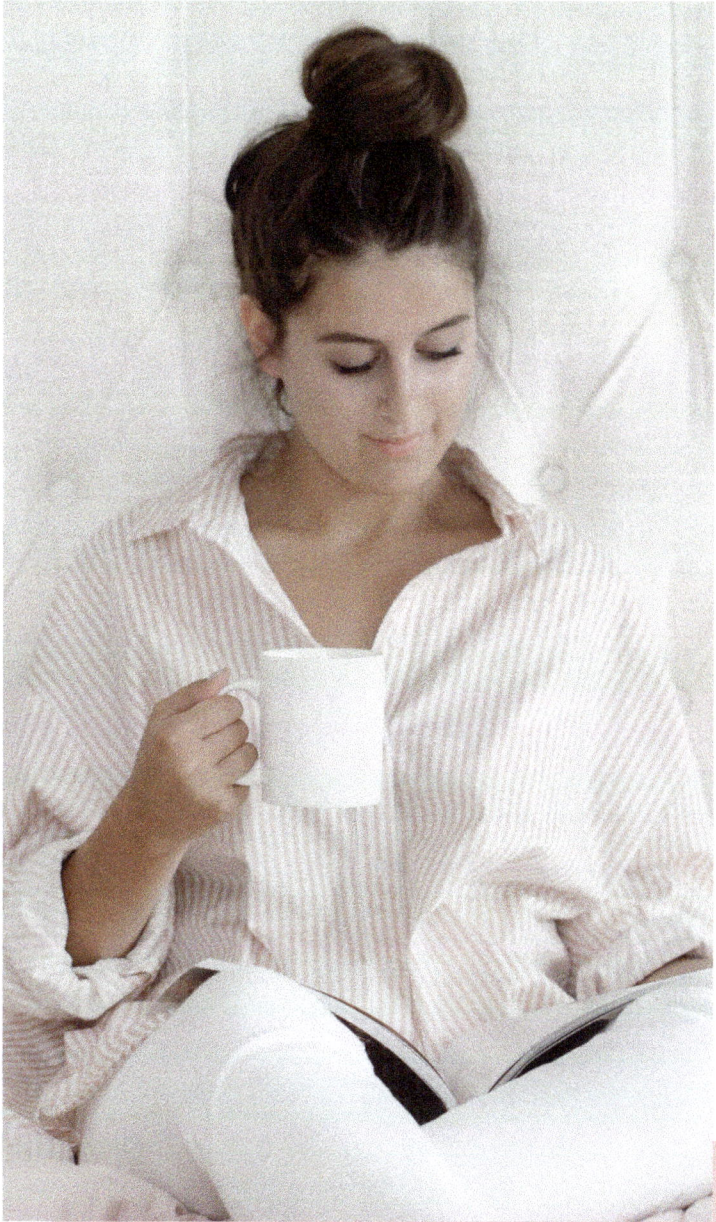

SLEEP
AND THE BODY

Sleep is vital to our health. Just as eating a healthy diet and exercising is important, we also need adequate rest to recuperate and help our body rebuild and repair tissue. Not sleeping enough doesn't just make you feel groggy the next day, it can affect how your brain functions while you're awake. There are several health problems linked to sleep deprivation.

WHAT DOES THE BRAIN DO WHILE WE SLEEP?

You may have thought that sleep was just a way to pass the time between midnight and 7 am, but it is much more than that. When we sleep, our brains are busy learning and growing, and the body is rebuilding and repairing itself at a time when it needs the least amount of energy.

CELL REPAIR AND RENEWAL

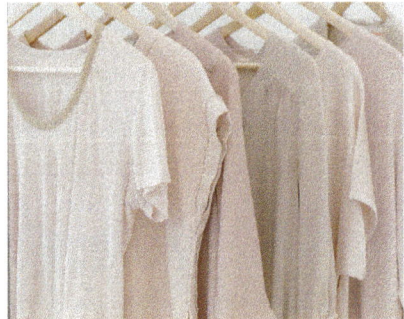

Several biological processes happen during sleep: the body repairs cells and tissue, and the brain communicates with nerve cells to store and organize information more efficiently. Everything the body can use gets assimilated, and what is left over is collected as waste. It's a very efficient system.

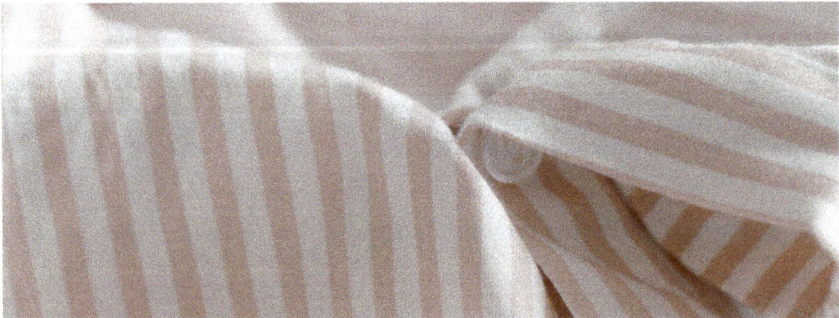

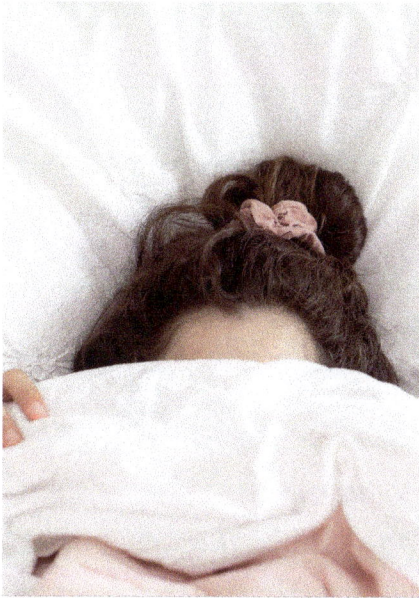

REST AND RECOVERY

While you sleep, your brain goes over all the day's events, storing information and memories and organizing everything for a clear, fresh start in the morning. When you get restful sleep, eight or more hours per night, the body can shut down specific systems, allowing them to rest and recuperate while repairing and restoring other systems to full functionality. The body needs this break at night to function in a healthy manner.

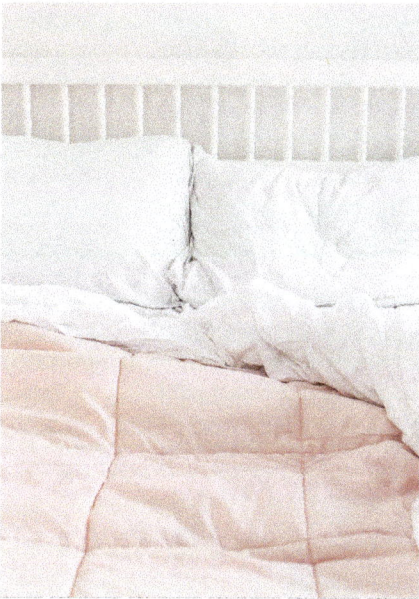

When the body is at rest, it experiences different levels of relaxation that allow the mind and body to rest completely. If we don't sleep long enough, these processes don't have time to do their magic, and things can quickly go downhill. People who work long hours often get in the habit of sleeping fewer hours to be more productive during the day. This can have a harmful effect on your central nervous system after a while.

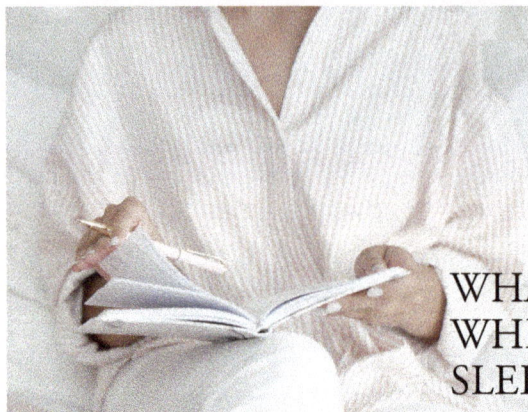

WHAT HAPPENS WHEN YOU DON'T SLEEP ENOUGH?

It is recommended that healthy adults sleep at least seven to eight hours per night, children need 12 to 14 hours, and infants the most in the first few months of life. Children need sleep because their bodies are still growing and developing, and adults need sleep for healthy brain function and cell repair. As we age, it requires more energy for the body to do what it needs to do.

Adults need sleep for healthy brain function and cell repair.

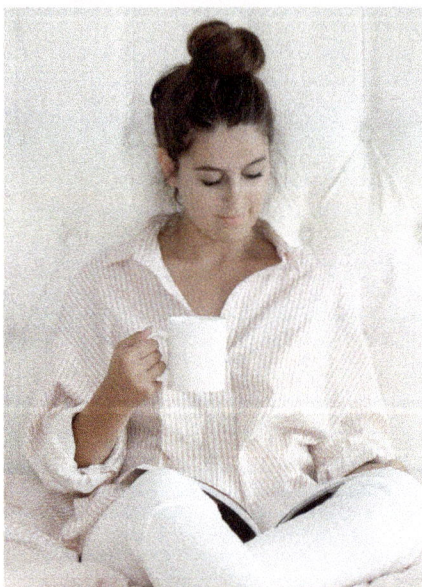

Due to hectic school schedules, demanding work schedules, and family obligations, many adults don't get the sleep their body needs. Having a new baby in the house, children who frequently wake during the night, and frequent bouts of insomnia can leave a person feeling weak and tired during

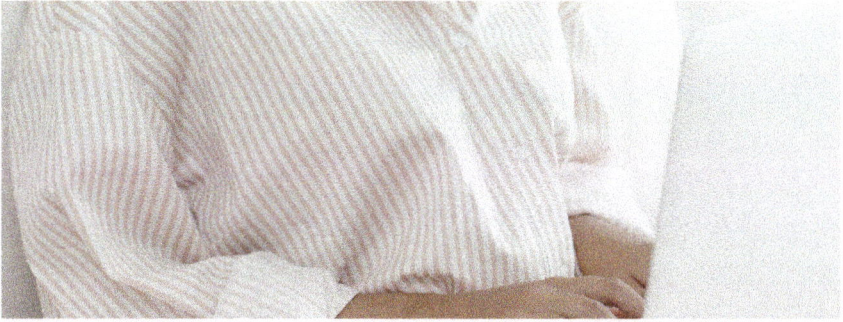

the day. Evening screen time can interfere with our normal sleep patterns since we tend to consume caffeine late at night, work on computers, and watch television.

Because restorative sleep is necessary for essential processes in the body, not getting enough rest can pose health risks. Lack of sleep for extended periods (sleep deprivation) can impact our thinking and influence our emotions, behavior, and decision-making abilities. In children, it can affect their ability to learn and make completing tasks difficult. When multiple parts of the body systems are affected by a lack of sleep, the person's overall health is at risk.

Sleep deprivation influences reaction time, which can be critical for driving safely. Every year, thousands of accidents are caused by drowsy drivers, resulting in serious injury and death. Transport companies require their drivers to sleep a certain number of hours daily, and they must pull over and stop until that time has passed. It is essential for the employee's health and the public's safety. Many highway deaths have been prevented with this requirement since drivers must comply with it.

Besides the usual daytime sleepiness caused by not sleeping at night, the individual may experience behavior changes or mood swings caused by irritability. It can also affect the immune system, causing the body to get overwhelmed and vulnerable to invading germs.

CHANGING YOUR SLEEP HABITS TO IMPROVE YOUR HEALTH

You see how the lack of restful sleep can affect the brain, body, and central nervous system. But, just the opposite, it can also make a significant impact. Changing your sleeping habits can improve your health by ensuring that the body has enough restful, restorative sleep to repair itself and fuel the system processes for healthy heart and brain function, immune system health, and hormonal balance.

Getting enough sleep every night is difficult for some people. It's not just a question of going to bed early enough. Not being able to shut down the brain and body for sleep means that you lie there tossing and turning, unable to fall asleep as you should.

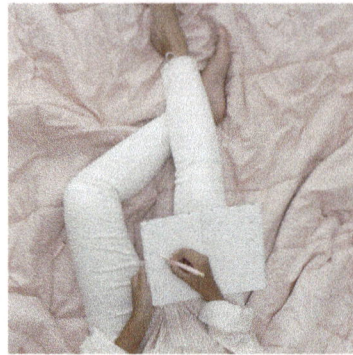

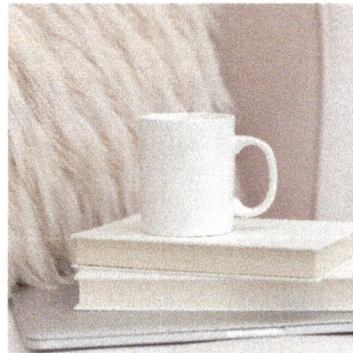

Changing your sleeping habits can improve your health by ensuring the body gets enough restful, restorative sleep to repair itself.

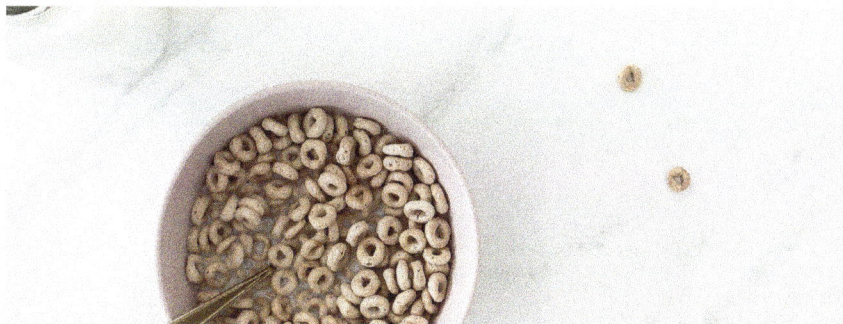

HELPFUL SUGGESTIONS

- Eat a well-balanced diet.
- Get adequate amounts of exercise daily.
- Take a warm shower or bath before bed.
- Make sure the room is at a comfortable temperature.
- Your mattress should be supportive and comfortable.
- Sleep with pillows to support your head and neck.

ESSENTIAL OILS CAN HELP YOU RELAX AND GO TO SLEEP

Besides the suggestions above, many things can help or promote falling asleep. But everyone is different, and what works for one person might not work for another. Essential oils have been around for thousands of years as a remedy to calm and soothe the body and mind. They have been used to help people relax and fall asleep naturally.

The chemical makeup of these essential oils makes them perfect for inducing restful relaxation. Each oil has its own properties, different from the others, which works for certain people, which means that everyone can find an oil that works best for them. You can experiment with different oils and mix and match them to your preferences. When it comes to sleep hygiene, everyone has their own sleep rituals, and essential oils are a perfect ingredient to add to your nightly routine to help you relax and sleep like a baby.

"*DEAR SLEEP, I'M SORRY WE BROKE UP THIS MORNING. I WANT YOU BACK!*"

– ANONYMOUS

CHAPTER FOUR

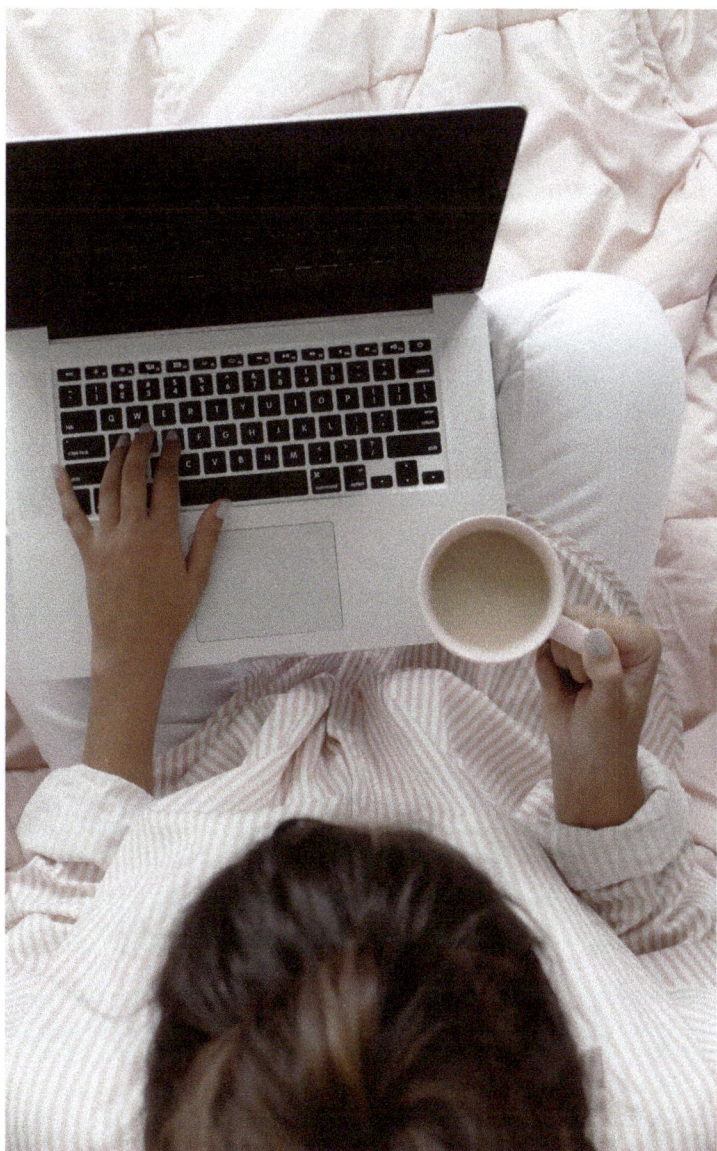

WHAT IS AN ESSENTIAL OIL?

Before examining how essential oils can help encourage sleep, let's first look at what an essential oil is and how it works. Essential oils are fragrant, vital fluids distilled from flowers, shrubs, leaves, trees, roots, and seeds. Because they are necessary for the life of the plant and play a vital role in the biological processes of the vegetation, these substances are called "essential." They carry the lifeblood, intelligence, and vibrational energy that endow them with the healing power to sustain their own life—and help the people who use them.

Essential oils come from aromatic plants and their parts, including trees, grasses, fruit, leaves, flowers, bark, needles, roots, and seeds. All essential oils have unique medicinal properties, characteristics, and therapeutic benefits that will differ depending on the soil, climate, and altitude of the countries where the plants were grown.

Plant substances extracted into essential oils are used in aromatherapy to promote well-being and good health. While the term aromatherapy can seem ambiguous, "scent" is only one aspect of aromatherapy, as you will discover many more dramatic benefits for healing the body, mind, and spirit.

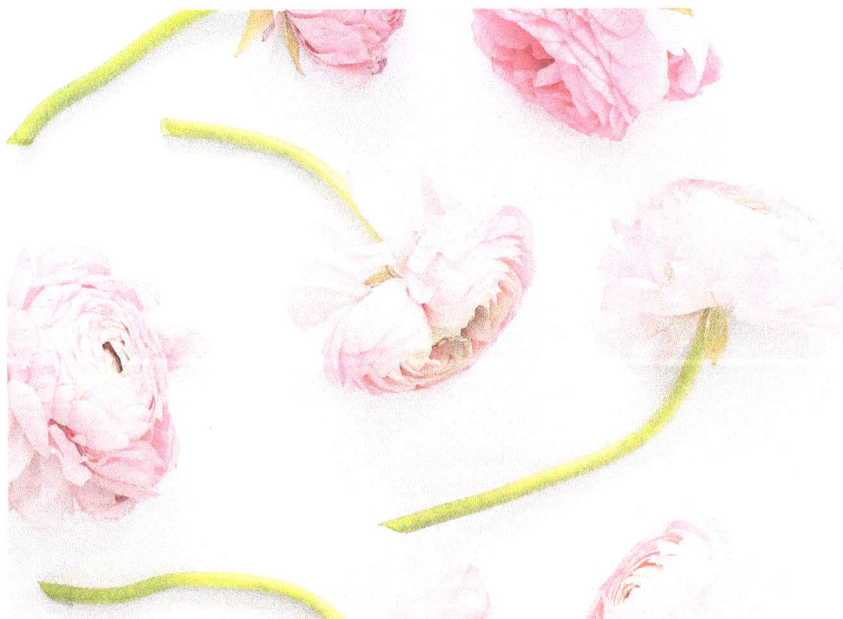

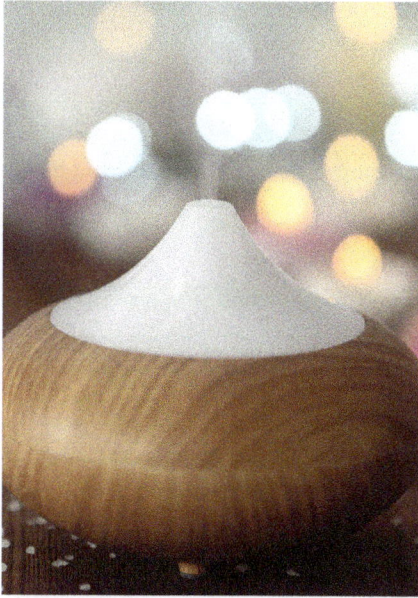

HOW ESSENTIAL OILS WORK

When essential oils are diffused in the air, the nose, wired differently than the other four senses, carries the oil's molecules directly into the head via the olfactory system. The olfactory membranes, with almost 800 million nerve endings, receive the micro-fine, vaporized oil particles and carry them along the axon of the nerve fibers, connecting them with the secondary neurons in the olfactory bulb. The sense of smell facilitated through the olfactory nerve invites the fragrance of essential oils into some areas of the brain, which enables the body to process them naturally. The scent molecules stimulate the brain's limbic region, pineal gland, and pituitary gland. Of the five human senses, the sense of smell is the only one that is directly connected to the brain.

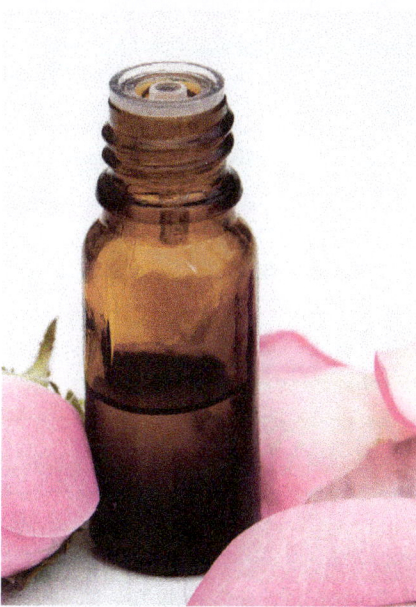

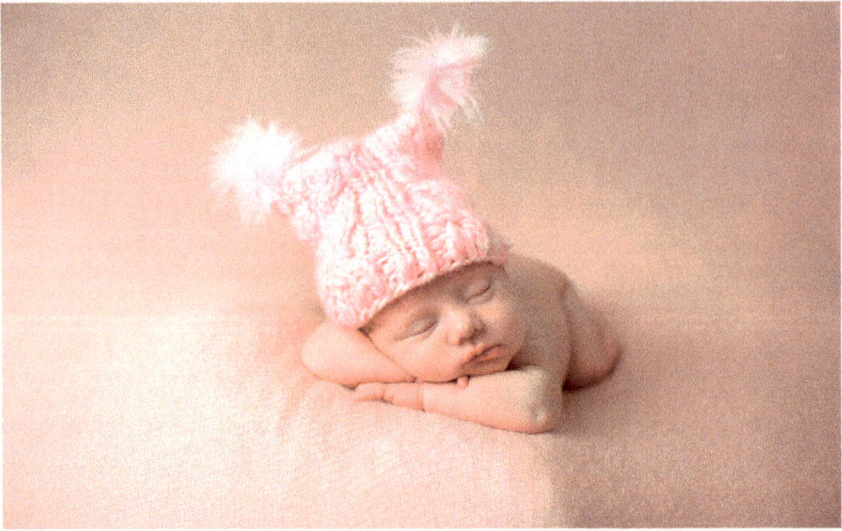

The olfactory system, closely linked to the limbic system, dramatically influences the body's physiology. Research has shown that these aromatic compounds can exert strong effects on the brain, especially on the hypothalamus (the hormone command center of the body) and the limbic system (the seat of emotions). Molecules that pass through the blood-brain barrier and stimulate various constituents of the brain can exert their effect quickly and result in pain relief and sleep promotion. This knowledge has been used to treat multiple conditions, such as sleep disorders and anxiety, and to provide relief for chronic pain.

The limbic system, which is directly linked to those areas of the brain that control our memory, blood pressure, heart rate, hormone balance, breathing, and stress levels, can be significantly influenced by essential oils, which can reach the limbic system by bypassing the cerebral cortex. This is important in that once inhaled, they affect the physiological and psychological function of the body with positive results. Therapeutic properties beneficial for the limbic system include antidepressant, calming, grounding, relaxing, and sedative.

OTHER METHODS

Certain essential oils can not only aid in sleep through their aroma but can also be applied topically or taken internally to promote restful sleep. When taken internally, these oils can help to calm the nervous system and promote relaxation. For example, Lavender oil can be used to promote peaceful sleep and ease feelings of tension. Similarly, Copaiba oil can be taken internally to help soothe and calm the nervous system. When using an essential oil topically, you will benefit from the aroma of the blend as well as the absorption through the skin.

Since everyone has different sleep patterns, preferences, and needs, each person will react differently to an essential oil and which method suits them. This makes essential oils especially good at promoting a restful environment, as you will find various methods and oils that suit you and your sleeping needs. If you find that one method doesn't create a relaxing atmosphere as you'd hoped, you can try another to see if it's a better fit for you.

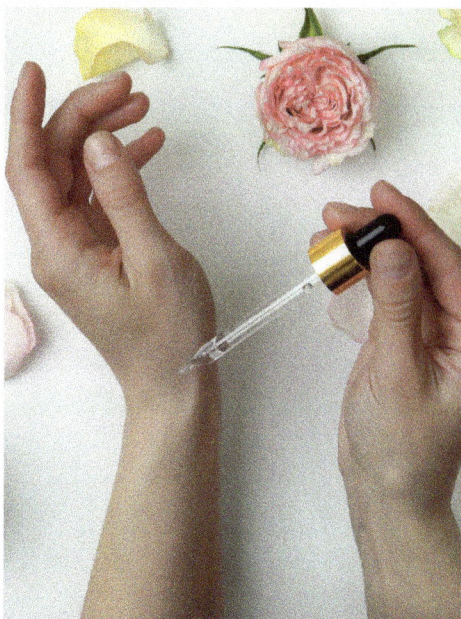

WHEN TAKEN INTERNALLY, CERTAIN OILS CAN HELP TO CALM THE NERVOUS SYSTEM AND PROMOTE RELAXATION.

"I'M SO GOOD
AT SLEEPING
THAT I CAN DO
IT WITH MY
EYES CLOSED."

– ANONYMOUS

CHAPTER FIVE

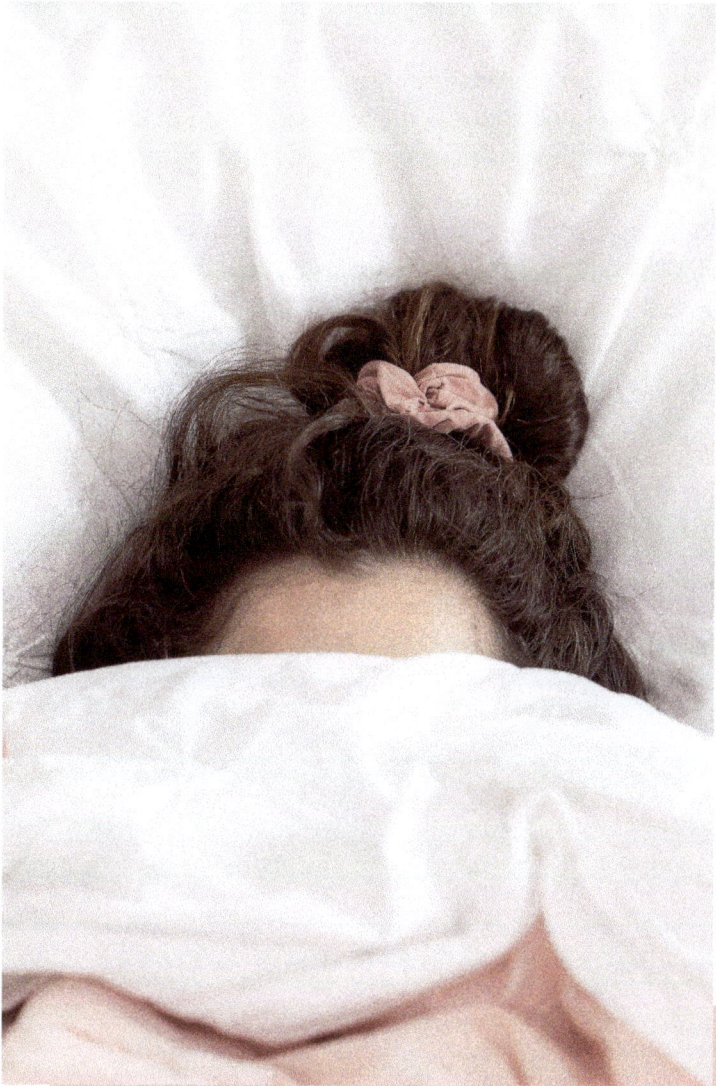

ESSENTIAL OILS GOOD FOR SLEEP

ESSENTIAL OIL PROPERTIES
BENEFICIAL FOR SLEEP

It's important to educate yourself and learn about each essential oil's unique properties and benefits when trying to pick suitable oils for bedtime. The goal is to choose oils to help create a calm, tranquil, and relaxing environment. Luckily, there are dozens of essential oils with aromas that can promote a restful atmosphere.

Before choosing an essential oil for sleep, we must first consider each oil's benefits, which will depend on its chemical components. Each essential oil has a unique chemical profile from any other oil in its group based on several factors, including the plant's part used for distillation and how it was distilled.

Depending on which part of the plant the oil is extracted from, some will have soothing properties, while others may be energizing and invigorating. To be suitable for sleep, an essential oil must have properties that are calming, soothing, and produce a relaxed state of being. This is the perfect environment needed for restful sleep.

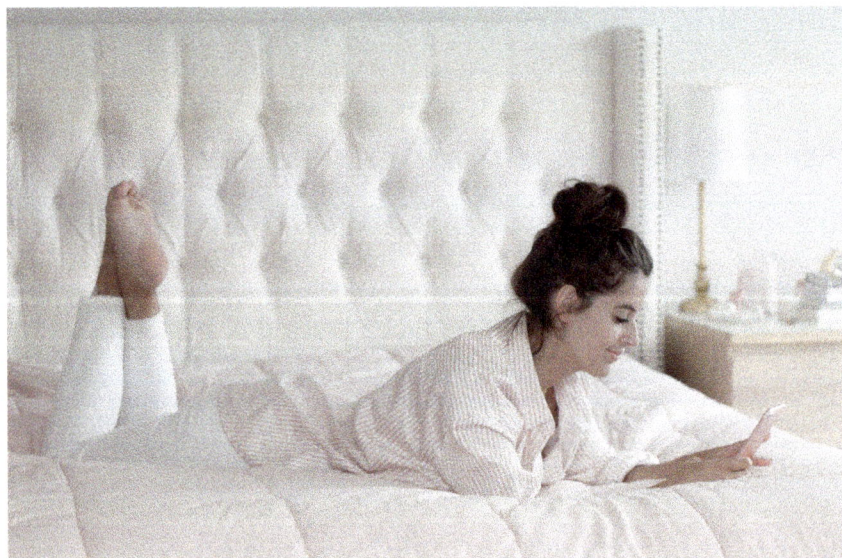

CALMING

Calming oils, consisting mainly of esters, can promote calm feelings for the body and mind. While the specific aromas listed below are very different, they produce similar effects in the body and can be used to promote calm feelings and relax the mind. Many essential oils considered beneficial for sleep possess calming therapeutic properties. Compounds like linalool and linalyl acetate, known for their relaxing properties, are abundant in essential oils like Lavender and Bergamot. These essential oils can be diffused in the bedroom to create a peaceful environment before bed. They can also be taken internally to calm the nervous system, promote relaxation, and lead to restful sleep.

- Lavender
- Clary Sage
- Petitgrain
- Roman Chamomile
- Bergamot
- Rose
- Orange
- Neroli
- Lemon
- Rose Geranium
- Helichrysum
- Jasmine
- Opoponax
- Rosalina

SOOTHING

Oils in the soothing category can be applied topically to soothe the skin and aromatically, at bedtime to soothe the body and the mind.

- Melissa
- Ylang Ylang
- Dill
- Benzoin
- Clary Sage

GROUNDING

Grounding oils are typically composed of alcohols or ketones and can help settle the body and mind before bed by promoting calm feelings.

- Cedarwood
- Sandalwood
- Vetiver
- Spikenard
- Ylang Ylang
- Cypress
- Galbanum
- Patchouli
- Valerian

HARMONIZING

These essential oils promote harmony and balance to help the body and mind prepare for a night of tranquil sleep. These oils are mainly composed of alcohols and can help encourage serenity to help you relax and sleep peacefully.

- Cilantro
- Marjoram
- Frankincense

WARMING

Warming oils can be used topically or aromatically before sleep to help promote calm, relaxed feelings. They often have a spicy aroma and feel warm on the skin. Remember to dilute warming oils before applying them to your skin, as they can be quite strong.

- Thyme
- Clove
- Black Pepper
- Cardamon
- Ginger
- Marjoram

SEVERAL BENEFITS AT ONE TIME

Because of their unique characteristics, an essential oil may be warming, soothing, invigorating, and calming, depending on its specific combination of chemical components. This means that one oil can have several valuable benefits.

With time and practice, you will find that each essential oil creates a different reaction within the body or brain. As you experiment with other oils and various application methods, these reactions can help you select your favorite essential oils for promoting relaxation and sleep. You can also combine several essential oils to help create a calm, relaxed feeling to help you relive stressful feelings, relax, and fall asleep.

It's about creating an environment that promotes a good night's sleep. You have many oils to choose from, and once you've found an essential oil with relaxing, calming, or soothing properties, you can incorporate it into your bedtime routine to help you sleep better at night.

Create your own scents by experimenting with and blending different oils to get the desired outcome.

After choosing the essential oils you want to use, decide which application (aromatically, topically, or internally) would give you the best results and allow you to get the rest you need.

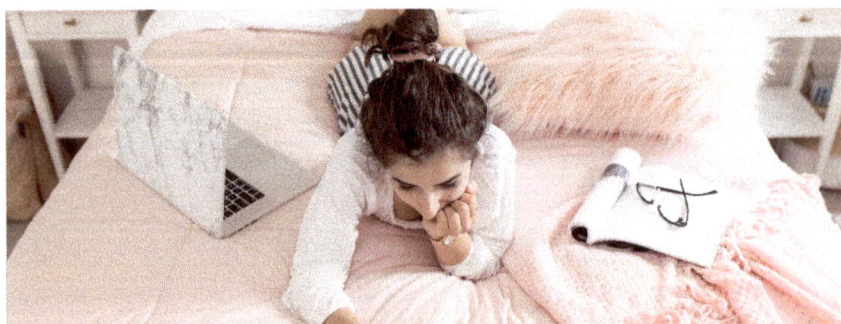

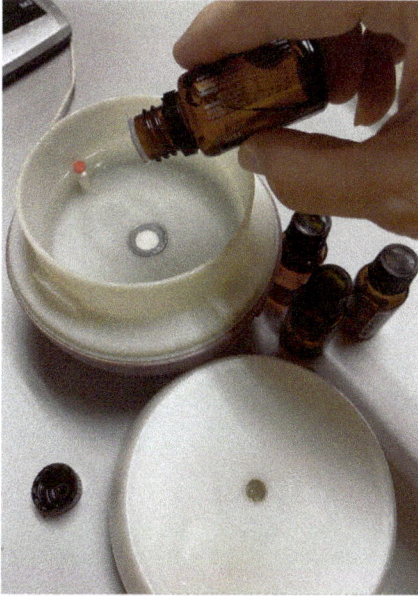

One of the best ways to experience the benefits of essential oils is to use a diffuser. This is a great way to enjoy the benefits of the oils before bedtime or when falling asleep. An essential oil diffuser in your bedroom permits you to breathe in the tranquil scent of the oil while you fall asleep. Mix a few drops of different essential oils together to create your bedtime diffuser blends.

You can mix a few calming oils with other essential oils you like to make a unique aroma that will help you create a calming environment that promotes sleep. But remember, not all oils you use in a diffuser have to fall within the "relaxing" or "calming" category.

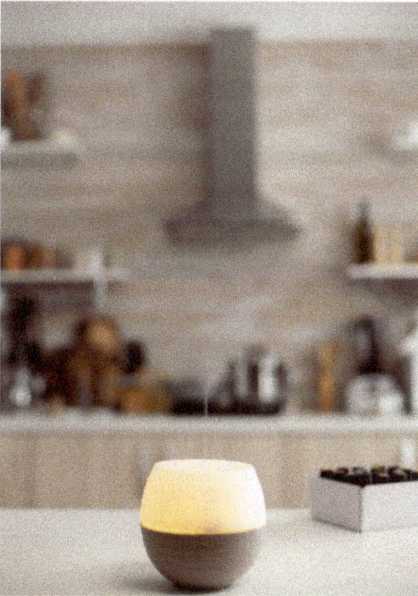

WHICH CHEMICAL COMPONENTS PROMOTE SLEEP?

Essential oils contain different properties, such as alcohols, esters, and ketones. Each of these components determines the oils' purpose and usefulness. Alcohols are composed of hydrogen and oxygen molecules, making them suitable for cleansing the skin, protecting against germs, supporting the heart, and inducing relaxing sleep.

Essential oils with alcohols that promote sleep include Clary Sage, Sandalwood, and Lavender.

Essential Oils that have ketones include Lavender and Dill.

Oils with a chemical group known as esters have a calming effect on mood. These include Roman Chamomile, Bergamot, Clary Sage, and Lavender.

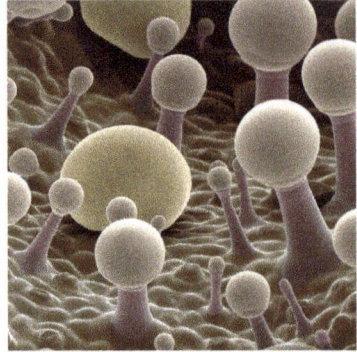

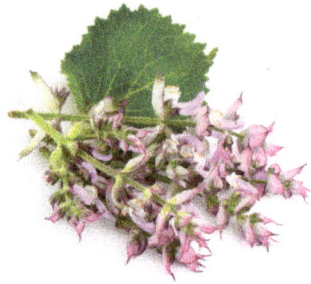

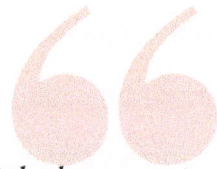

Oils that contain the chemical group esters have a calming effect on mood.

HOW A CHEMICAL COMPONENT
MAKES IT USEFUL FOR SLEEP

When essential oils are inhaled, molecules from the essential oils make their way to the brain, where they affect the amygdala.

Essential oils via the olfactory system cause the brain to secrete neurotransmitters, such as dopamine and serotonin, which can elevate a person's mood. These neurotransmitters make you feel calm and relaxed. Serotonin is needed to produce melatonin, the hormone responsible for making you feel sleepy at bedtime.

Essential oils that contain chemical properties with a soothing, calming, or relaxing nature induce a positive response within the brain and the body.

After inhaling an essential oil with calming properties, the brain processes the aroma, and a physical effect follows afterward.

The brain then positively associates and makes a connection with this aroma and, from then on, recognizes it. Using this particular oil with the calming property for sleep can continue to be used because of this connection between the fragrance and the brain.

Everyone has different preferences, needs, and sleep patterns and will react differently to an essential oil. This is what makes it so helpful in promoting an environment conducive to sleep. If one essential oil doesn't promote quality sleep like you hoped it would, you can try another one with similar components known to help with sleep and see if it is a better fit.

WHICH OILS HELP SUPPORT GOOD SLEEPING HABITS?

It is best to choose essential oils with chemical constituents that provide soothing, calming, and relaxing benefits for the body, mind, and mood. You can experiment with different ones to see which specific oils best fit your needs and preferences when promoting sleep.

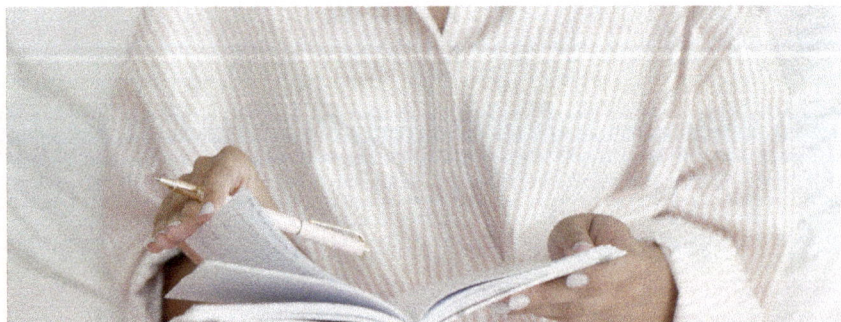

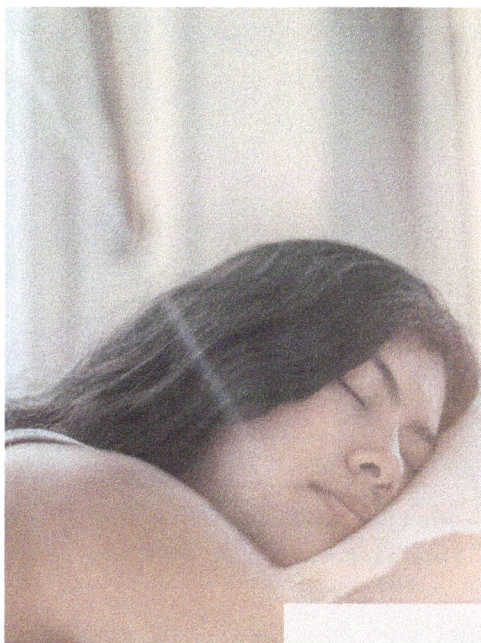

HOW TO CHOOSE AN ESSENTIAL OIL TO HELP YOU SLEEP

Doing a little research and learning about the benefits of each essential oil will help you narrow down your choices for finding an essential oil for sleep. You will want to choose oils that promote deep feelings of relaxation. Combining the following oils with a sleep routine that supports healthy sleep will have a positive effect.

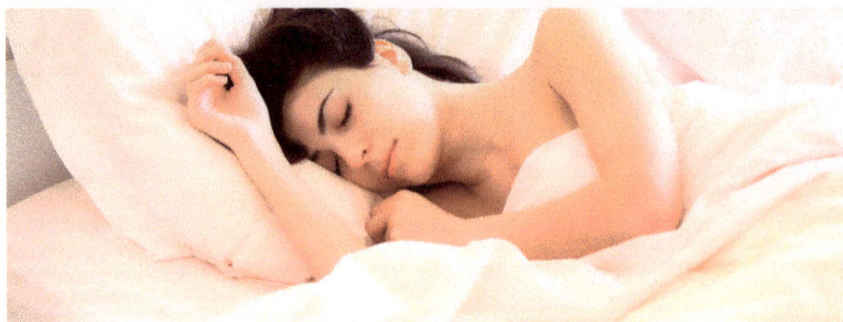

ESSENTIAL OIL BENEFITS

The essential oils listed below interact with the brain and body differently. Each oil possesses characteristics that promote sleep, making it easy to find an oil that works for you.

Bergamot used before bedtime helps promote a sense of calm and harmony.

Cedarwood oil allows the mind and body to unwind before retiring for sleep.

Cilantro oil promotes a peaceful feeling, supporting a restful night's sleep.

Clary Sage oil has a relaxing, balancing nature that can help create a restful environment for sleep.

Lavender oil used aromatically is perfect for creating an environment conducive to sleep.

Frankincense oil has a soothing aroma that can help induce feelings of peace and relaxation.

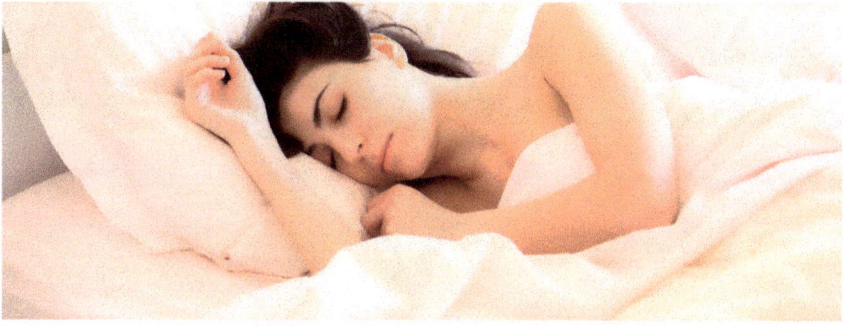

ESSENTIAL OIL BENEFITS

To see which oils work best for you in promoting good sleep, keep it simple by choosing essential oils known for their relaxing properties.

- Melissa oil calms tense feelings and can be used at nighttime to promote deep relaxation.

- Marjoram oil has calming properties to help lessen stress.

- Petitgrain oil helps promote restful sleep by promoting feelings of calmness and easing tension.

- Roman Chamomile oil has a calming effect on the body and quiets the mind.

- Ylang Ylang oil helps reduce the effects of stress while promoting a calming environment.

- Sandalwood oil is good for promoting relaxation and deep sleep.

"SANDALWOOD OIL IS GOOD FOR PROMOTING RELAXATION AND DEEP SLEEP."

CHAPTER SIX

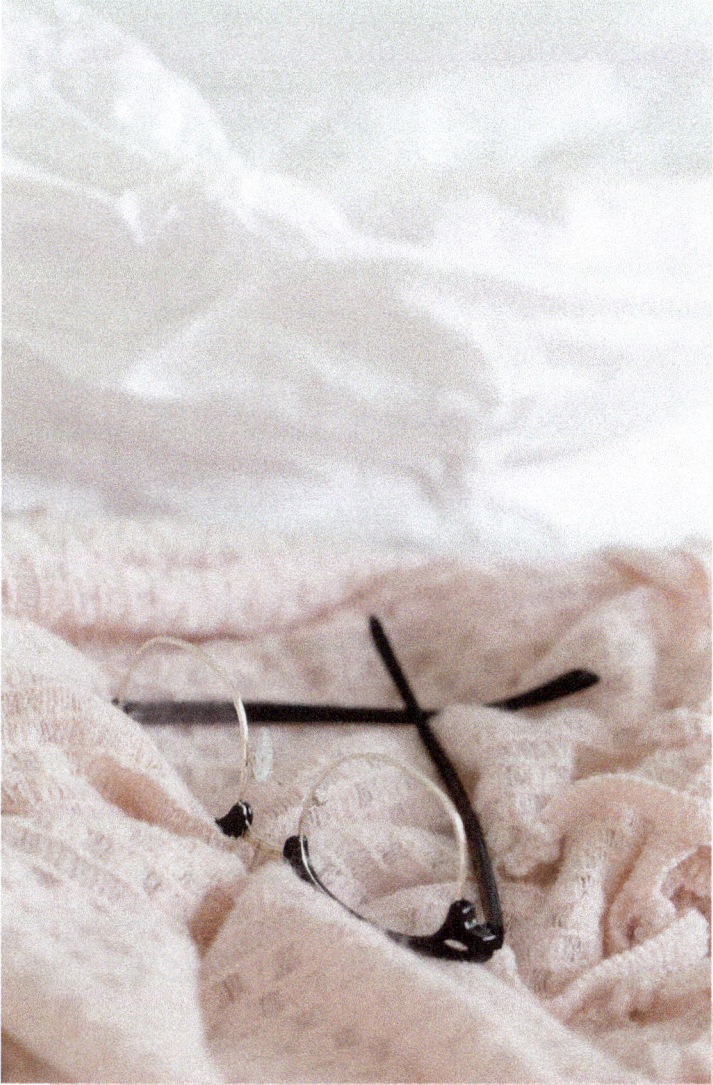

ESSENTIAL
OIL PROFILES

If you are already familiar with essential oils, you probably know of several oils that promote relaxation and may help you get into a restful state, ready to sleep. Research supports that insomnia has been effectively treated with essential oils. Some studies have shown that Lavender is more effective in inducing sleep and relaxation than prescribed medication. Adding a few drops of a relaxing essential oil to a bedside diffuser is one of the most pleasant ways to enhance the sleeping experience.

Specific essential oils smell nice, but they also train your mind to unwind and allow your body to relax and drift off to sleep. Try adding essential oils to your bedtime routine and train your brain to associate a specific scent with falling asleep.

Of course, essential oils are not a "magic pill." What may work for some people may be ineffective for you. This is because essential oils are adaptogens and affect people differently. Be flexible and try other oils until you find the best fit.

Certain essential oils are energizing and stimulating. You will want to avoid using these at bedtime. The best essential oils for insomnia are oils that are calming and reduce anxiety and stress. Government studies suggest that using essential oils before retiring can alleviate mild sleep disorders.

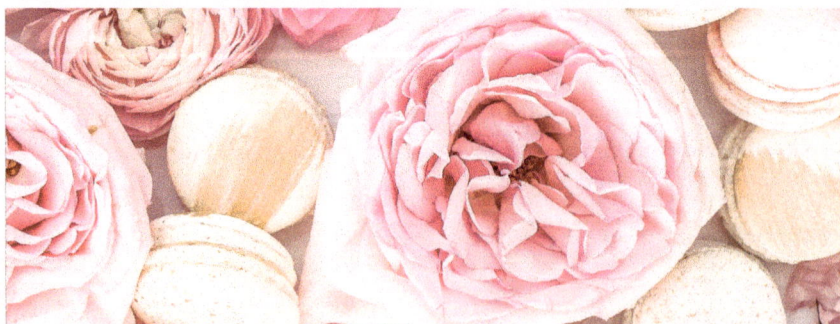

BERGAMOT

Bergamot is a favorite oil for aromatherapists in treating depression. Bergamot is an antispasmodic and that helps to reduce leg cramps and is used for restless leg syndrome. Studies have shown that bergamot oil can reduce anxiety and improve mood. Better yet, Bergamot essential oil is thought to reduce the presence of cortisol in saliva, which gives it its sedative properties. Those with sleep apnea may want to try it to keep breathing evenly through the night. The therapeutic properties of Bergamot include analgesic, antidepressant, antiseptic, antibiotic, antispasmodic, stomachic, calmative, cicatrisant, deodorant, digestive, febrifuge, vermifuge, and vulnerary. Unlike many other citrus oils that can be energizing, Bergamot is calming, reduces stress and anxiety, and possesses sedative qualities. It has been used for centuries to aid digestion and is thought to help maintain neural pathways in the brain. Research has also indicated that Bergamot can ease chronic pain. Bergamot lowers your heart rate and blood pressure, helping with anxiety and stress, and allowing you to get to sleep. Bergamot's sedative property helps the body relax and heal. Its antispasmodic property helps calm the muscles while increasing blood flow and circulation to promote a quicker healing time. Bergamot essential oil has phototoxic properties. Therefore, exposure to the sun must be avoided after use. It may also interfere with the activity of certain prescription drugs (NSAIDs, proton-pump inhibitors, acetaminophen, antiepileptics, immune modulators, blood-sugar medications, blood pressure medications, antidepressants, antipsychotics, diabetic medications, antihistamines, antibiotics, and anesthetics).

Usage: oral, topical, inhalation

Note: top

CEDARWOOD

Cedarwood contains therapeutic properties that are anti-seborrheic, antiseptic, antispasmodic, anti-inflammatory, tonic, circulatory stimulant, antirheumatic, astringent, diuretic, emmenagogue, expectorant, insecticide, sedative and fungicidal. Like Lavender, Cedarwood is considered suitable for detoxifying and clearing negative emotions. Because inhaling Cedarwood triggers the release of serotonin in the brain, which converts to melatonin, the essential oil is known for its sedative qualities and usefulness in treating insomnia. Cedarwood has been shown to decrease heart rate and blood pressure, maintaining its usefulness as a sleep aid and alleviating hypertension and anxiety. Cedarwood essential oil has also been found to reduce involuntary motor activity and prolong sleep for those people with restless legs and other movements during the night. It is considered a non-toxic and non-irritant oil. It is a relaxing and soothing oil that allows the brain to stop processing.

Usage: topical, inhalation

Note: base

ROMAN CHAMOMILE

Roman Chamomile is another popular oil for insomnia. There are several species of chamomile, but Roman chamomile (*Anthemis nobilis aka Chamaemelum nobile*) essential oil is the most potent for battling insomnia. Roman Chamomile is an ancient herb with therapeutic properties, including sedative and relaxing. It is recommended to treat insomnia, stress, restless leg syndrome, and nervous tension, so it is an excellent choice to help you relax and prepare for sleep. Try combining Roman Chamomile essential oil with true Lavender essential oil for a more powerful treatment. The therapeutic properties of Roman Chamomile oil are analgesic, antispasmodic, antiseptic, antibiotic, anti-inflammatory, anti-infectious, antidepressant, antineuralgic, antiphlogistic, bactericidal, carminative, cholagogue, cicatrisant, emmenagogue, febrifuge, hepatic, sedative, nervine, digestive, tonic, sudorific, stomachic, vermifuge and vulnerary. It is non-toxic and non-irritant. Roman Chamomile's ability to act as a mild sedative to ease nerves and decrease anxiety to treat conditions like hysteria, nightmares, insomnia, and other sleep difficulties has also been researched. While the root of these effects is not determined, they appear to be psychological. Studies also have shown Roman Chamomile's effectiveness in relieving stress and anxiety. It has a warm, sweet, herbaceous scent that is relaxing and calming for both mind and body. Roman Chamomile's gentleness makes it especially valuable for restless children.

Usage: oral, topical, inhalation

Note: middle

GERMAN CHAMOMILE

German Chamomile is a relaxing and rejuvenating agent that calms nerves, reduces stress, and aids insomnia. German Chamomile is known for its anti-inflammatory abilities and can help alleviate muscle spasms and joint pain. Its therapeutic properties include analgesic, anti-allergic, anti-convulsive, antidepressant, antiseptic, antispasmodic, anti-inflammatory, cholagogue, diuretic, emmenagogue, febrifuge, hepatic, nervine, sedative, splenetic, stomachic, sudorific, tonic, vermifuge, and vasoconstrictor. Azulene gives this oil its intense blue color, while sesquiterpenes lend its calming effect. German Chamomile calms nerves, eases headaches, and aids in relaxation. It operates as a mild tranquilizer and as a sleep inducer. German Chamomile impacts the same areas of the brain and nervous system as popular anti-anxiety medications and can also assist in minimizing aches and pains. Its calming reputation and stress-reducing effects are due to apigenin, which German Chamomile contains and is known to bind to benzodiazepine receptors. Of course, the benefits of German Chamomile are not restricted to the use of its essential oil. The plant's flower can be enjoyed as a relaxing hot drink when brewed as a tea.

Usage: oral, topical, inhalation

Note: middle

CLARY SAGE

Clary Sage can be used as an antidepressant and as a sedative. Women experiencing hormonal changes or menopause symptoms such as hot flashes find this oil beneficial. Clary Sage's properties are antidepressant, anticonvulsive, antispasmodic, anti-inflammatory, antiseptic, aphrodisiac, astringent, bactericidal, carminative, deodorant, digestive, emmenagogue, euphoric, hypotensive, nervine, sedative, stomachic, uterine, and nerve tonic. Clary Sage oil is non-toxic and non-sensitizing. Its anti-inflammatory and antispasmodic properties help to calm and soothe the body and mind. It also aids in reducing pain associated with inflammation. Clary Sage is a natural sedative that may reduce your cortisol levels, known as the stress hormone. Do not use it during pregnancy or if you are at risk for breast cancer, as it may have an estrogen-like effect on the body. Clary Sage is similar to Valerian in that it affects the GABA receptors, which help reduce stress. Clary Sage also has mood-lifting properties that are useful in treating patients who suffer from depression. When this oil was compared to others, such as Chamomile and Lavender, it was the most effective at combating stress.

Usage: oral, topical, inhalation

Note: top-middle

CORIANDER

Coriander works as an analgesic, antirheumatic, antispasmodic, carminative, deodorant, fungicidal, revitalizing, and stimulating. It relieves mental fatigue, migraine pain, stress, and nervous debility. Coriander's warming effect helps alleviate pain such as rheumatism, arthritis, and muscle spasms. The healing properties of Coriander oil are attributed to phytonutrient content, including carvone, geraniol, limonene, borneol, camphor, elemol, and linalool. Coriander is traditionally used in India for its anti-inflammatory properties. Coriander oil is also beneficial for removing heavy metals and toxins from the body.

Usage: oral, topical, inhalation

Note: top

CYPRESS

Cypress is an incredibly gentle oil that calms and soothes anger while positively affecting one's mood. It assists with varicose veins and bodily fluids by improving circulation. Its properties include antibacterial, anti-infectious, anti-inflammatory, anti-rheumatic, antiseptic, antispasmodic, astringent, decongestant, diuretic, and vein tonic. Avoid use during pregnancy. It may interact with aspirin, blood pressure, antiplatelet, and anticoagulant medications.

Usage: topical, inhalation

Note: middle-base

DILL

Dill is a stimulating, revitalizing, restoring, purifying, and balancing oil. Dill oil, when used aromatically, can help lessen stress and reduce anxious feelings. This oil can be used internally before bed to help promote restful sleep. Its healing properties include antispasmodic, carminative, digestive, disinfectant, galactagogue, sedative, stomachic and sudorific. Dill helps relieve cramps, diarrhea, flatulence, and indigestion. Dill Seed is non-toxic and non-irritating. Avoid use during pregnancy.

Usage: oral, topical, inhalation

Note: middle

FRANKINCENSE

Frankincense is highly prized in the aromatherapy industry as a potent anti-inflammatory with sedative properties. Frankincense helps reduce inflammation's pain while calming the body and mind and promoting healing. The therapeutic properties of Frankincense oil are antiseptic, astringent, antirheumatic, antispasmodic, carminative, cicatrisant, cytophylactic, digestive, diuretic, emmenagogue, expectorant, sedative, tonic, uterine, vulnerary and expectorant. Frankincense may promote relaxation to calm you, helping you to fall asleep. Frankincense is known to send messages to the limbic system that help to reduce stress and improve mood. It can also help to reduce anxiety and relieve pain and inflammation. Frankincense essential oil helps open passageways, which can help reduce snoring and allow your body to take deep, calming breaths. This oil is non-toxic, non-irritant, and non-sensitizing. Frankincense can be inhaled, applied topically, or ingested.

Usage: oral, topical, inhalation

Note: base

JASMINE

Jasmine is well respected for its aphrodisiac properties and is a sensual, soothing, calming oil that promotes love and peace. In another 2010 study, Jasmine was as effective for calming nerves as a sleeping pill or sedative drug except without side effects. It is important to note that all absolutes are extremely concentrated by nature. The complexity of the fragrance, particularly the rare and exotic notes, is well regarded as an aphrodisiac. However, it is also considered an antidepressant, antiseptic, cicatrisant, expectorant, galactagogue, parturient, sedative, uterine and antispasmodic. Jasmine has been known to assist with restless sleep, thereby enhancing your sleep quality. Avoid use during the first and second trimesters of pregnancy.

Usage: topical, inhalation

Note: base

LAVENDER

Lavender (*Lavandula angustifolia*) is an effective essential oil to help you fall asleep and stay asleep. Lavender is predominately made up of alcohols and esters and has several therapeutic properties, many associated with relaxation. Lavender is the most popular essential oil, but be aware that several species, such as Spike Lavender (Lavandula latifolia) and the hybrid Lavandin (Lavandula x intermedia), have very similar properties but are not as sedating as true Lavender. Lavender is known to improve sleep quality, increase the time spent in deep, slow-wave sleep, and relieve restlessness and negative emotions.
In one study, people who had inhaled Lavender oil the night before reported feeling more "vigorous" the next day, confirming that they had received additional restorative slow-wave sleep.
In another study, the use of Lavender among individuals with insomnia found that it led to improved sleep quality and that women and younger volunteers with milder insomnia enjoyed even more significant benefits. Lavender is known to calm anxiety and offers sedative effects. Not only does it help you to fall asleep, but Lavender helps you to spend more quality time in deep, slow-wave sleep. Research revealed that a Lavender foot bath could improve blood flow and encourage changes in the autonomic nervous system often seen when people are relaxed. Applying some of this oil to the body diluted in a carrier oil before bed at night may also be effective.

Usage: oral, topical, inhalation

Note: middle

LAVANDIN

Lavandin properties include analgesic, anticonvulsive, antidepressant, antiphlogistic, antirheumatic, antiseptic, antispasmodic, antiviral, bactericidal, carminative, cholagogue, cicatrisant, cordial, cytophylactic, decongestant, deodorant, and diuretic. It is considered one of the most valuable and versatile essential oils, from easing sore muscles and joints, relieving muscle stiffness, clearing the lungs and sinuses from phlegm to healing wounds and dermatitis. Its analgesic properties aid in alleviating pain. Its calming scent reduces anxiety and promotes sleep. This oil is non-toxic, non-irritating, and non-sensitizing. Caution when used during pregnancy.

Usage: topical, inhalation

Note: middle

LEMON

Lemon is recognized due to its refreshing and cooling properties. It is suitable for the circulatory system and aids blood flow, reducing blood pressure. Citral, myrcene, and limonene, all present in citrus oils, have been shown in some studies to lengthen sleep duration and relax muscles. Lemon's therapeutic properties are anti-anemic, antimicrobial, anti-rheumatic, anti-sclerotic, antiseptic, bactericidal, carminative, cicatrisant, depurative, diaphoretic, diuretic, febrifuge, hemostatic, hypotensive, insecticidal, rubefacient, tonic and vermifuge. Lemon is non-toxic but could cause skin irritation for some. It is also phototoxic and should be avoided before exposure to direct sunlight.

Usage: oral, topical, inhalation

Note: top

LEMONGRASS

Lemongrass is known for its stimulating qualities and makes an excellent antidepressant. This essential oil promotes blood circulation by dilating the blood vessels, allowing uninterrupted blood flow. Lemongrass helps reduce inflammation. It has potent analgesic and anti-inflammatory properties. Lemongrass not only tones but fortifies the nervous system and can be used in the bath for soothing muscular nerves and pain with its potent analgesic and anti-inflammatory qualities. This oil relieves the symptoms of jet lag, helps with nervousness and anxiety, and clears headaches. The therapeutic properties of Lemongrass oil are analgesic, antidepressant, antimicrobial, antipyretic, antiseptic, astringent, bactericidal, carminative, deodorant, diuretic, febrifuge, fungicidal, galactagogue, insecticidal, nervine, nervous system sedative and tonic. Avoid use with individuals with glaucoma. Use caution in prostatic hyperplasia and with skin hypersensitivity or damaged skin. Safe for topical and ingestion if appropriately diluted.

Usage: oral, topical, inhalation

Note: top

LEMON MYRTLE

Lemon Myrtle is a highly potent antibacterial and germicide that is a much more effective germ killer than Tea Tree. It is beneficial for colds, flu, chest congestion, cold sores, warts, irritable digestive problems, flatulence, and skin conditions. This oil improves concentration, relaxation, and better sleep when diffused in the air.

Usage: topical, inhalation

Note: top

LINALOE BERRY

Linaloe Berry properties include anti-allergenic, anti-anxiety, antidepressant, antihistamine, anti-infectious, anti-inflammatory, antispasmodic, calming, sedative, tonic, and support the immune system. It promotes sleep and assists with pain caused by injury or muscle soreness. This oil is considered non-irritating and non-sensitizing for most.

Usage: topical, inhalation

Note: middle

MANDARIN

Mandarin is often used as a digestive aid and to ease anxiety. This tangy oil increases circulation to the skin and reduces fluid retention. Mandarin therapeutic properties include antiseptic, antispasmodic, cytophylactic, depurative, sedative, stomachic, and tonic. Direct sunlight should be avoided after use, as it may be phototoxic.

Usage: oral, topical, inhalation

Note: top

MARJORAM SWEET

Marjoram Sweet (*Origanum marjorana*) essential oil is the only Majoram recommended for helping with insomnia due to its calming and sedating action on the nervous system, which is known to lower blood pressure, ease nervous tension and hyperactivity, and soothe loneliness, grief, and rejection–all of which can exacerbate insomnia. Sweet Marjoram's sleep-inducing effects are thought to be even more effective than those of Lavender and Chamomile; both are used more often as sleep aids. Like Lavender, Marjoram produces a highly effective synergistic blend for insomnia. Using Marjoram will undoubtedly give you a better night's sleep. Marjoram is a comforting oil that can be massaged into the affected area or added to a warm compress to ease discomfort. It helps treat tired, aching muscles when used in a sports massage blend. Marjoram's pain-relieving properties are helpful for rheumatic pains, sprains, spasms, swollen joints, and achy muscles. Marjoram is superb as a relaxant and is helpful for headaches, migraines, and insomnia. Marjoram's therapeutic properties are analgesic, antispasmodic, antiarthritic, antirheumatic, anaphrodisiac, antiseptic, antiviral, anti-inflammatory, bactericidal, carminative, cephalic, cordial, diaphoretic, digestive, diuretic, emmenagogue, expectorant, fungicidal, hypotensive, laxative, nervine, sedative, stomachic, vasodilator, and vulnerary. Its sedative properties allow the body to heal, reduce inflammation and eliminate pain. Marjoram is generally non-toxic, non-irritating, and non-sensitizing.

Usage: oral, topical, inhalation

Note: middle

MAY CHANG

May Chang, also known as *Litsea cubeba*, has properties that include antifungal, antiviral, antiseptic, antimicrobial, and anti-inflammatory. This oil helps with insomnia and soothes aches and pains. It may irritate the skin and mucous membranes. May Chang could increase pressure on the eyes, so avoid using it if you suffer from glaucoma.

Usage: topical, inhalation

Note: top

MELISSA

Melissa, also called Lemon Balm, is well known for its uplifting properties. Its healing properties include being antidepressant, anti-inflammatory, antiviral, antispasmodic, bactericidal, carminative, cordial, diaphoretic, emmenagogue, nervine, sedative, stomachic, sudorific, and tonic. Melissa has strong sedative qualities and treats emotional trauma and shock. It is considered non-sensitizing and non-toxic. Please check with your healthcare provider before use during pregnancy.

Usage: oral, topical, inhalation

Note: middle-top

NEROLI

Neroli is used for its relaxing and slightly hypnotic effects, and it can also help with lucid dreaming and spark creativity. It aids sleep due to its soothing qualities and functionality as a natural tranquilizer. One study found that Neroli oil, in combination with Lavender and Chamomile oil, was effective in reducing anxiety, increasing sleep, and stabilizing blood pressure. Another study revealed that Neroli could reduce postmenopausal symptoms, increase sexual desire, and reduce blood pressure in postmenopausal women. Neroli is also known to help relieve muscle spasms and heart palpitations. Neroli's therapeutic properties are antidepressant, antiseptic, anti-infectious, antispasmodic, aphrodisiac, bactericidal, carminative, cicatrisant, cytophylactic, cordial, deodorant, digestive, sedative, and tonic. This oil is non-toxic and non-sensitizing.

Usage: topical, inhalation

Note: middle-top

OPOPONAX

Opoponax, also known as Sweet Myrrh, properties include analgesic, antifungal, anti-anxiety, antibacterial, anti-inflammatory, antiseptic, astringent, antispasmodic, calming, and carminative, disinfectant, emmenagogue, expectorant, immune stimulant, stomachic, sedative, tonic, and vulnerary. This oil is helpful for menopause. Topically this oil may be used similarly to Myrrh in balms, ointments, and salves. It is also beneficial for relaxing muscles, reducing stress, and treating anxiety. It may be phototoxic; therefore, avoid direct sunlight for 12 hours. Avoid use during pregnancy.

Usage: topical, inhalation

Note: base

PATCHOULI

Patchouli is beneficial for combating nervous disorders and nausea, treating depression, and reducing fever. This oil's therapeutic properties include antidepressant, anti-inflammatory, antimicrobial, antiseptic, antitoxic, antiviral, aphrodisiac, astringent, bactericidal, deodorant, diuretic, fungicidal, nervine, prophylactic, stimulating, and tonic agent. As a sedative oil, it allows the body to relax and rest, allowing healing to begin. It may interact with aspirin, blood pressure, antiplatelet, and anticoagulant medications and increase the risk of bleeding among people with bleeding disorders.

Usage: oral, topical, inhalation

Note: base

PETITGRAIN

Petitgrain is believed to have uplifting properties and is used for calming anger and stress. Petitgrain is valued for its ability to reduce pain and spasms in the lower intestines. Its calming qualities make it a favorite for insomnia. This oil's properties include antidepressant, antiseptic, antispasmodic, deodorant, immuno-support and stimulant, tonic, and sedative for the nervous system. Petitgrain is generally considered non-toxic, non-irritant, and non-sensitizing.

Usage: oral, topical, inhalation

Note: top

ROSALINA

Rosalina is well known for its antiseptic, spasmolytic, and anticonvulsant properties. Rosalina has anti-infectious properties and helps to relax and calm individuals who may be stressed deeply. It is helpful for insomnia and other sleep disorders. Rosalina's therapeutic properties include antibacterial, antimicrobial, analgesic, anti-anxiety, cicatrisant, immunostimulant, antiviral, anti-inflammatory, and mucolytic. Avoid use during pregnancy.

Usage: topical, inhalation

Note: middle

ROSE GERANIUM

Rose Geranium has the ability to both uplift and sedate. It is considered a wonder oil for emotions and balances the hormonal system. Rose Geranium is non-toxic, non-irritant, and generally non-sensitizing, though it can cause sensitivity in some people. Its therapeutic properties include antidepressant, anti-inflammatory, antiseptic, astringent, antispasmodic, cicatrisant, emmenagogue, and sedative. Avoid use during pregnancy.

Usage: oral, topical, inhalation

Note: middle

ROSE

Rose is an uplifting aphrodisiac and is excellent for meditation. Rose oil treats depression, grief, anger, and other unpleasant emotions. It supports the heart and is considered one of the most amazing remedies for female problems, such as balancing hormones during menopause. It helps to reduce muscle spasms and pain from injury and inflammation. The therapeutic properties of Rose are antidepressant, antiphlogistic, antiseptic, antispasmodic, antiviral, aphrodisiac, astringent, bactericidal, choleretic, cicatrisant, depurative, emmenagogue, hemostatic, hepatic, laxative, nervous system sedative, stomachic and a tonic for the heart, liver, stomach, and uterus. Rose oil relieves pain by activating the TRPV1 receptor (a sensor that detects pain). Avoid use during the first trimester of pregnancy.

Usage: oral, topical, inhalation

Note: base

ROSEWOOD

Rosewood is credited as being a bactericidal, antifungal, antiviral, antiseptic, antispasmodic, anti-parasitic, cellular stimulant, immune system stimulant, tissue regenerator, tonic, antidepressant, antimicrobial, analgesic, bactericidal, cephalic, sedative, and an aphrodisiac. It is also regarded as a general balancer of emotions and helps with insomnia. Rosewood is rich in linalool, a chemical that can be transformed into several derivatives of value to the flavor and fragrance industries. It is a possible irritant to sensitive skin. Avoid use during pregnancy.

Usage: topical, inhalation

Note: base

SANDALWOOD

Sandalwood is known to create an exotic, sensual mood with a reputation as an aphrodisiac. In aromatherapy, it has been used for years to reduce and relieve inflammation. Sandalwood is used to reduce swelling and muscle spasms by inhibiting the 5-lipoxygenase (5-LOX) enzyme that is involved in the inflammation response. Its sedative effect allows the body to relax and heal. Sandalwood is used to help combat mood disturbances and stress. Santalol, a major component of Sandalwood oil, has been found to have a depressive effect on the central nervous system, enabling users to get more sleep. In sleep-disturbed rats, it causes a significant decrease in total waking time and an increase in total non-rapid eye movement sleep, which is the deepest type of sleep. Sandalwood's therapeutic properties are antiphlogistic, antiseptic, antispasmodic, astringent, carminative, diuretic, emollient, expectorant, sedative, and tonic. Sandalwood can aid in relaxation and calm anxiety. It is also known to have sedative effects. Sandalwood is considered non-toxic, non-irritant, and non-sensitizing.

Usage: oral, topical, inhalation

Note: base

SPIKENARD

Spikenard is used by aromatherapists for rashes, wrinkles, cuts, insomnia, migraines, and wounds. It brings peaceful tranquility. This oil's therapeutic properties are anti-inflammatory, antifungal, antispasmodic, sedative and tonic. Spikenard should be avoided during pregnancy.

Usage: oral, topical, inhalation

Note: base

VALERIAN

Valerian is used to combat insomnia, nervousness, restlessness, tension, agitation, panic attacks, and headaches resulting from nervous tension. It has also been used on muscle spasms, heart palpitations, cardiovascular spasms, and neuralgia. Valerian is a suitable replacement for catnip based on similar chemical components and is gaining popularity as a natural alternative to commercially available sedatives. The therapeutic properties of Valerian are antispasmodic, bactericidal, carminative, diuretic, hypnotic, hypotensive, regulator, sedative, and stomachic. It has possible skin-sensitizing properties, though it is non-toxic and non-irritating at low doses. Avoid use during pregnancy and with children. Valerian has been shown to reduce anxiety, which can help you to fall asleep and stay asleep longer and improve the quality of your sleep. It is calming to the nervous system and helps with restlessness. Valerian essential oil contains valerenic acid. According to a study published in the US National Library of Medicine National Institute of Health, valerenic acid is known to help subjects get better sleep. It helps people to fall asleep easier, get deeper and more restorative sleep, and decreases the number of times people wake up in the middle of the night.

Usage: oral, topical, inhalation

Note: base

VETIVER

Vetiver is profoundly relaxing and comforting. Its calming and soothing effect helps to relieve and reduce symptoms of inflammation. It helps to promote circulation and reduce pain. This oil helps dispel irritability, anger, and hysteria while having a balancing effect on the hormonal system. It is relaxing to the nervous system and helps with overstimulation. Vetiver oil's therapeutic properties are antiseptic, aphrodisiac, cicatrisant, nervine, sedative, tonic, and vulnerary. There is no known toxicity.

Usage: oral, topical, inhalation

Note: base

VIOLET LEAF

Violet Leaf is known for being relaxing, soothing, and inspiring absolute. It can treat stress, headaches, nervousness, insomnia, rheumatism, poor circulation, and sore throats. This oil is considered non-toxic and non-irritating but may cause sensitization in some individuals.

Usage: topical, inhalation

Note: base-middle

YLANG YLANG

Ylang Ylang assists with problems such as high blood pressure, rapid breathing, heartbeat, nervous conditions, impotence, and frigidity. The therapeutic properties of Ylang Ylang are antidepressant, antiseborrheic, antiseptic, aphrodisiac, hypotensive, nervine, and sedative. Ylang Ylang helps balance both sides of the brain and aid in the processing and releasing of negative emotions, like anger. Ylang Ylang oil can be combined with Bergamot oil to help reduce blood pressure, pulse, stress, anxiety, and cortisol. When it comes to sleep, Ylang Ylang can help you fall asleep faster while lowering stress and anxiety. Ylang Ylang is also a sedative and can have calming effects in relieving anxiety. Ylang Ylang may cause sensitivity in some people, and excessive use may lead to headaches and nausea. This oil is not recommended if you have low blood pressure. Ylang Ylang is a great oil to use for falling asleep if you find your mind racing in the day's activities and you struggle to settle it.

Usage: oral, topical, inhalation

Note: base

CHAPTER SEVEN

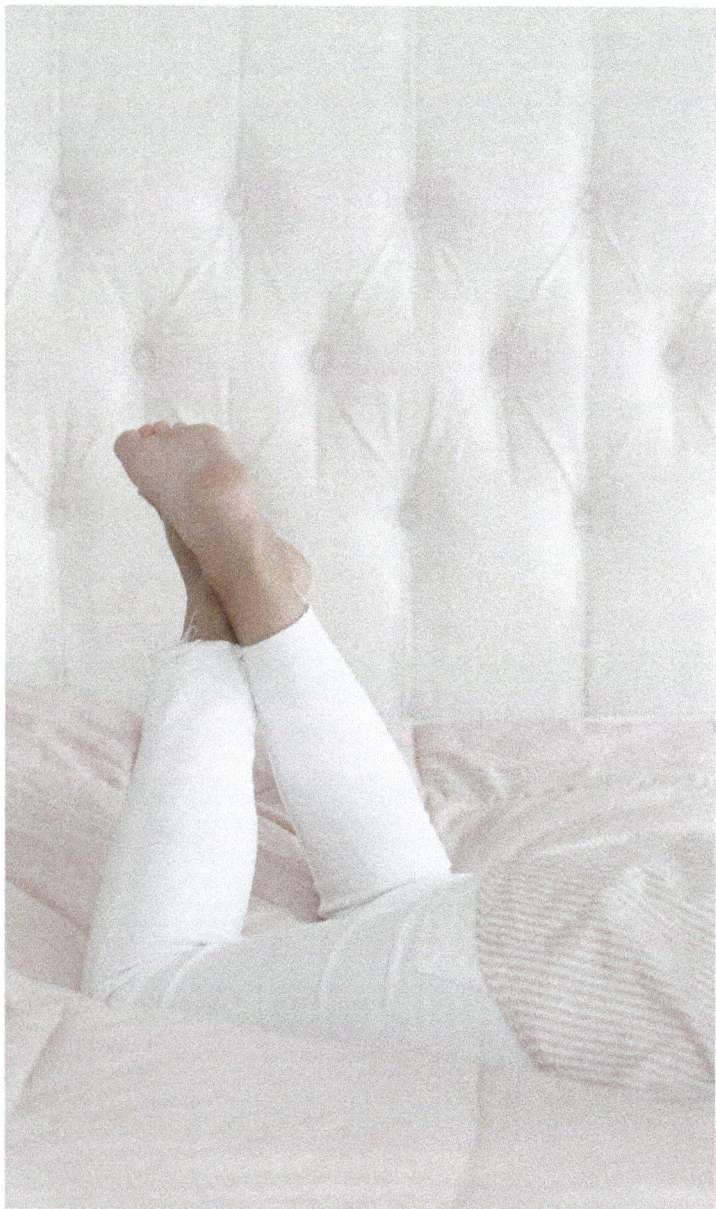

HOW TO USE ESSENTIAL OILS FOR SLEEP

Incorporating essential oils and natural remedies such as aromatherapy and relaxation techniques into your life can be very beneficial for some health conditions. When used correctly, most essential oils are safe and free of adverse side effects. However, as with any substance you introduce into your body, it is necessary to use them intelligently.

Most essential oils that have sedative or relaxing qualities may be used to help bring some relief to insomnia. If you know the underlying cause of your insomnia, you might find additional essential oils you can combine in a blend with the oils suggested. For example, you may want to combine Bergamot (*Citrus bergamia*) or Sweet Orange (*Citrus sinensis*) in a depression-related insomnia blend since these essential oils uplift the emotional system while relaxing the body.

While many people with sleep loss can benefit from certain essential oils, there are some factors you must take into consideration.

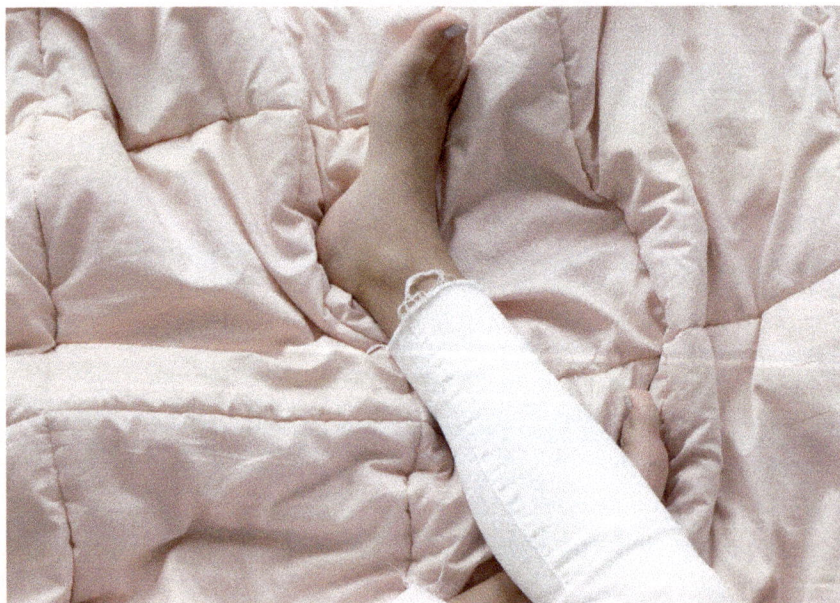

ESSENTIAL OIL USAGE FACTORS

Dosage – Dose is the most significant factor in essential oil usage. Some essential oils used in the wrong doses, such as in too high of a concentration, have been found (in animal and laboratory studies) to cause adverse effects on the body. Some essential oils can damage the skin, liver, and other organs if misused.

Quality – The purity of the essential oil is important. Even when oil is labeled as pure, it may be adulterated with added synthetic chemicals or similar smelling, cheaper essential oils or vegetable oil. Make sure your oils are of therapeutic quality.

Application – An essential oil that is safe when applied in one way may not be safe when used in another way. Some oils are considered safe if inhaled and yet may be irritating if applied to the skin in concentration. For instance, citrus oils such as

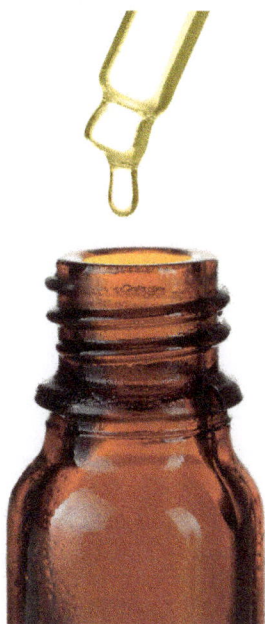

DOSE IS THE MOST SIGNIFICANT FACTOR IN ESSENTIAL OIL USAGE.

Bergamot and Lemon can cause phototoxicity (severe burn to the skin) if a person is exposed to the sun after topical application. However, this would not result from inhalation.

Lifestyle – Insomnia is a debilitating health condition. It is important to combine your use of essential oils with diet and lifestyle changes to achieve success with your natural remedy.

Drug Interaction – If you're currently under a doctor's care, talk to your doctor before starting any treatment program with essential oils. You will want to ensure that your oils will not interfere with the prescribed medications.

Another option is to find a naturopath to talk about holistic health care. This person will look at your health as a whole instead of treating symptoms of individual conditions. As you study and research therapeutic quality essential oils, you will find these are a great way to complement your whole-body care instead of taking a handful of pills daily for multiple medical issues.

Tip: The suggestions for essential oils in this book are for you to use as complementary care to the healthcare plan you already have. You may need to change your diet and other lifestyle modifications for all things to work together. If you do not achieve satisfactory results in improving sleep, please seek professional medical help.

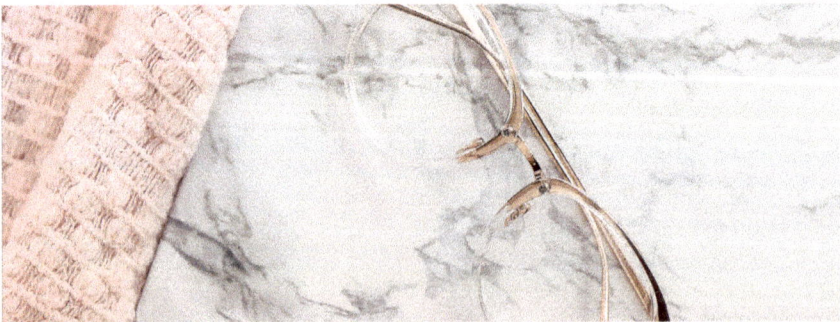

METHODS OF USE

Incorporating essential oils and natural remedies such as aromatherapy and relaxation techniques into your life can be very beneficial for insomnia. When used correctly, most essential oils are safe and free of adverse side effects. However, as with any substance you introduce into your body, there are some factors you must take into consideration.

Several options are available for treating sleeplessness in both allopathic and alternative medicine. Many people today can improve their sleep quality with the help of therapeutic quality essential oils along with vigilance and commitment to a healthy diet and lifestyle.

Various mechanisms can be used to deliver essential oils to target sites in the body. Typical routes of administration include inhalation, topical, and ingestion. Regardless of which route of administration is used, the essential oils have to travel to the site of action with either the help of blood, nerves, or oxygen (when the inhalation route is used). Combining these three approaches will ensure success.

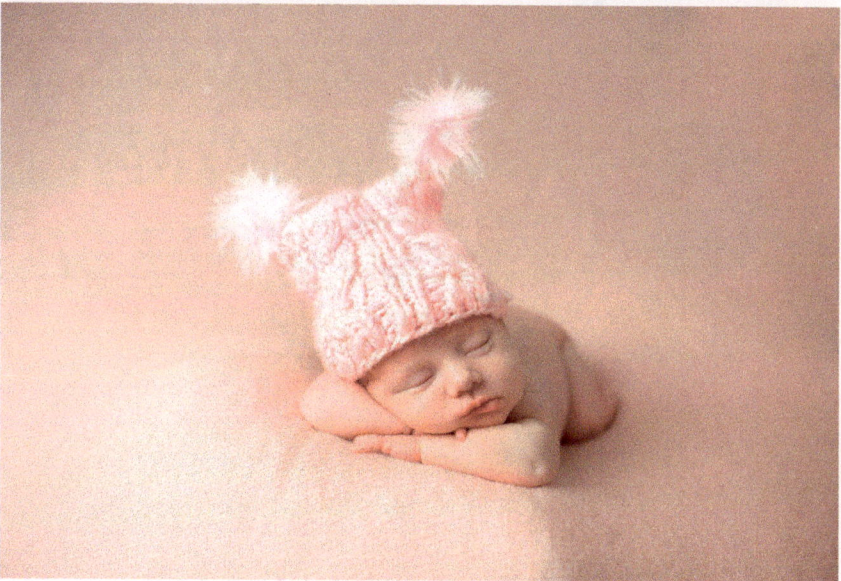

"LAVENDER ENHANCES SLEEP QUALITY BY INCREASING TIME IN DEEP SLOW-WAVE SLEEP."

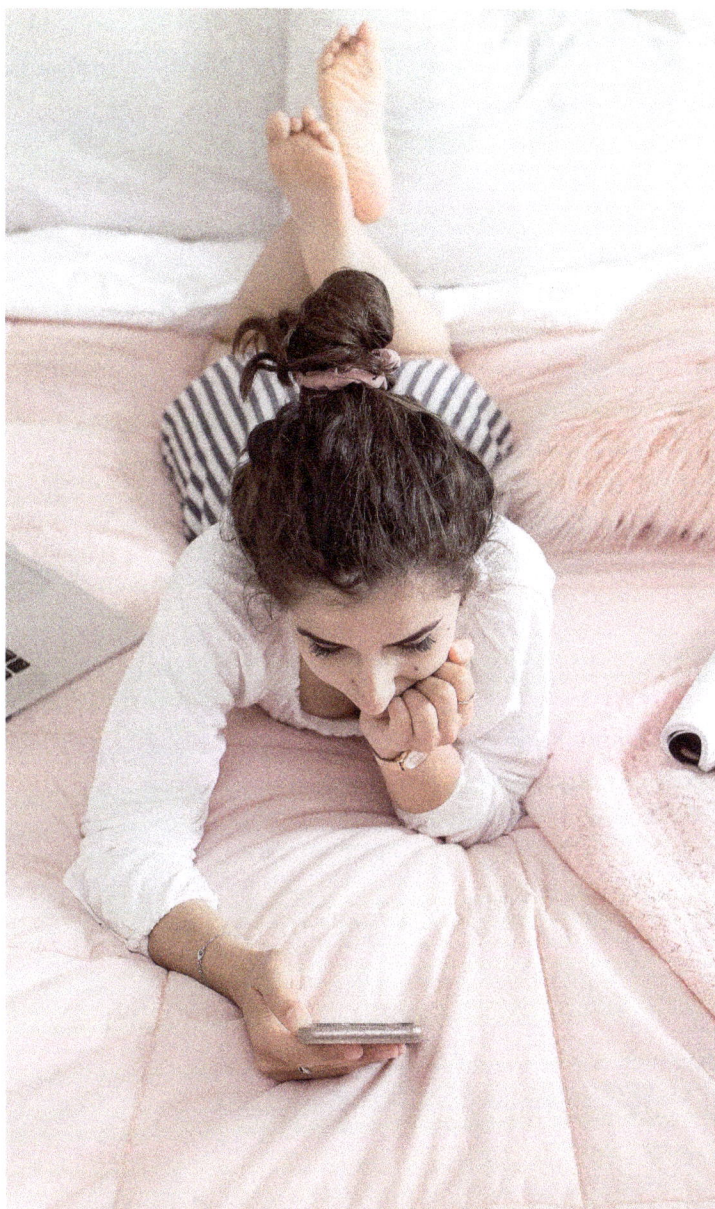

CHAPTER EIGHT

AROMATIC USE

Inhalation is one of the most natural methods of use and is considered the most direct pathway for an aromatic blend or essence. When inhaled, fragrant vapors enter the lungs and are instantly released into the bloodstream for delivery to every cell in the body. Scientific research shows that essential oils can remain in a person's bloodstream for up to 4-6 hours, depending on the essential oil.

Essential oils that are adequately diffused are known to improve mental clarity, enhance or calm emotions, and increase feelings of well-being. If a diffuser is not available, making a room spray, personal inhaler, or placing a few drops on a tissue to inhale will suffice. All are very effective ways to benefit from the therapeutic properties of essential oils. For inhalation, use intermittent exposure (not more than 15 minutes in an hour).

Inhalation of certain essential oil vapors triggers the olfactory bulb, which immediately sends a neurochemical signal to neuro-receptors. For example, smelling Lavender essential oil triggers the release of serotonin from the raphe nucleus in the brain and produces a calmative effect. Essential oils can easily be absorbed via inhalation and enter the bloodstream to deliver healing constituents throughout the body. Inhalation presents the least amount of risk for most individuals.

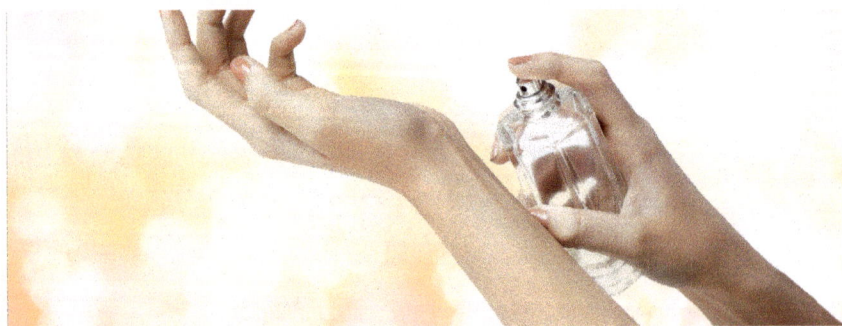

"DIFFUSING ESSENTIAL OILS IS KNOWN TO IMPROVE MENTAL CLARITY, CALM EMOTIONS, AND INCREASE FEELINGS OF WELL-BEING."

WAYS TO USE

01 DIFFUSER

Try adding essential oil or blend of choice to a diffuser. Use a nebulizer to diffuse your selection of oils for an hour, three times a day. You may want to use one specific essential oil, or you may blend a combination of essential oils. Place 10-12 essential oil drops into a diffuser in the bedroom and run for 15 minutes before bed.

02 CUP HANDS

Place 2-3 drops of your chosen essential oil in your hand and rub your palms together. Cup hands over your nose and inhale deeply. Or, smell from the bottle directly.

03 PERSONAL INHALER

Add 1-2 drops of essential oil to a tissue and carry with you to smell throughout the day, or add several drops of pure essential oil to a pocket diffuser and use 2-3 times daily.

04 ROOM SPRAY

Spritz your pillow and bedsheets with a relaxing room spray before bed. Choose a relaxing fragrance and use 10-15 minutes before bed.

WAYS TO USE

05 ## SMELLING SALTS
In a small tub or 10 ml (1/3 oz.) glass bottle, add 30 drops of the essential oil blend and fill the remainder of the bottle with either fine or coarse sea salt. Waft the bottle under your nose while taking deep breaths whenever you feel the need to shut your mind off and fall asleep.

06 ## SHOWER STEAMERS
Make these ahead and drop them in a hot shower or bath to relax. You can also add a few drops of a relaxing essential oil to Epsom salts for a nice bedtime bath.

07 ## COTTON BALL
Add a few drops to a tissue or cotton ball and tuck inside your pillowcase.

08 ## BOTTLE
Simply open the bottle and take a sniff several times before going to sleep.

"ADD A FEW DROPS TO A TISSUE OR COTTON BALL AND TUCK INSIDE YOUR PILLOWCASE."

DIFFUSER BLENDS

Pleasant, relaxing aromas used in a diffuser are one of the most effective ways to improve sleep. The diffuser transforms the oil into a fine mist of oil droplets which disperse the scent throughout the air. This enables you to enjoy its pleasing aroma for an extended period of time, making it the most convenient way to use essential oils for sleeplessness.

There are plenty of essential oil diffusers to choose from. Before buying one, evaluate your needs to determine which model will serve you best. Be sure the diffuser doesn't heat the oil as this may change its molecular structure, rendering it less potent and effective (glass nebulizer, waterless is best).

USING AN ESSENTIAL OIL DIFFUSER SAFELY

If you have other health conditions, you may want to consult with a certified aromatherapist before using essential oils aromatically to improve sleep. Essential oils can be highly potent, and reactions will differ from person to person.

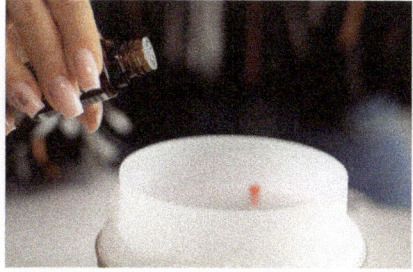

HOW TO CHOOSE AN ESSENTIAL OIL DIFFUSER

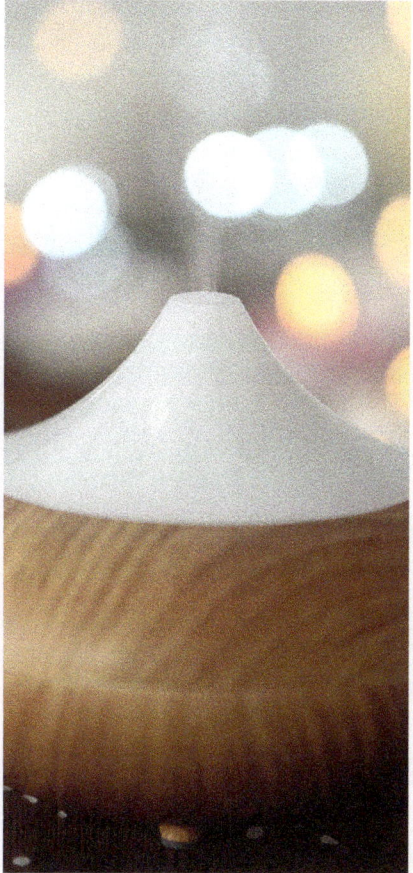

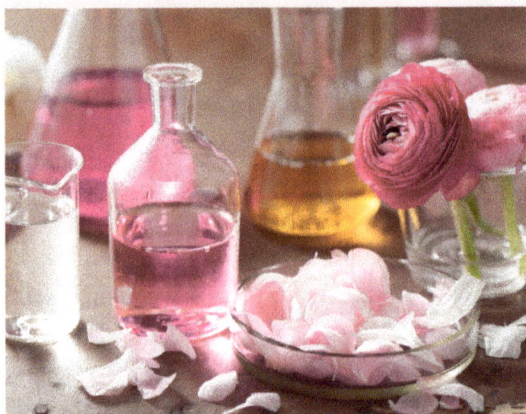

BLENDING ESSENTIAL OILS

Combining several essential oils in one diffuser is one way to enjoy the benefits of essential oil diffusion. Blending your diffuser blend creates a new aroma that is unique and different. The number of combinations you can make are limitless, but it might be difficult to know which oils pair well with others and which don't. For best results, follow the instructions below to learn how to make essential oil blends at home.

Combine several essential oils in your diffuser to enjoy the benefits of essential oil diffusion.

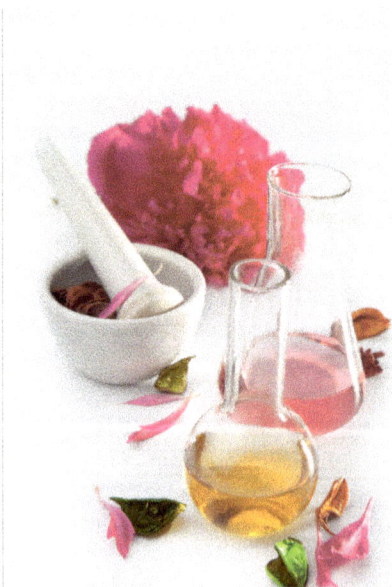

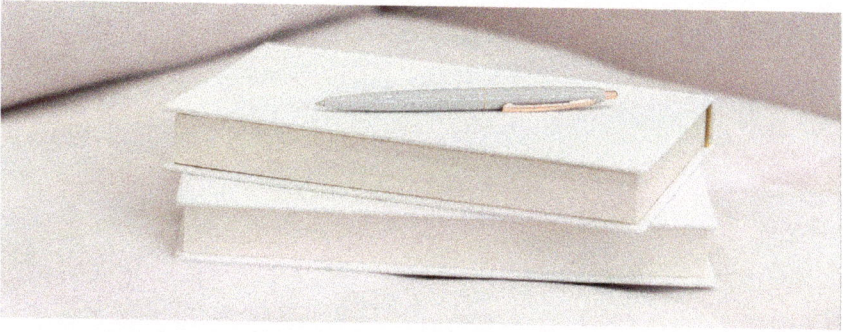

TIPS FOR MAKING A GOOD DIFFUSER BLEND

1. Determine the desired effect you want from the diffuser blend. The type of oil you use will determine the feeling you want to experience, such as relaxing, calming, or invigorating.
2. Are you trying to create a calming environment? Once you determine the desired outcome, choosing oils complementing one another will be easier.
3. Choose a group of oils with similar properties to help you achieve your desired effect. If you want a relaxing diffuser blend, choose oils known for calmness and serenity, like Lavender. Choose oils with stimulating properties like Peppermint or Lemon if you want an energizing effect.
4. Once you have decided on the oils you want to use, you can begin pairing them together.

Choose a group of oils with similar properties to help you achieve your desired effect.

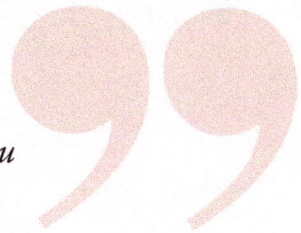

DIFFUSER BLEND RECIPES

SLEEP LIKE A BABY

3 drops Spikenard essential oil
3 drops Sweet Orange essential oil
2 drops Cedarwood essential oil

HIT THE SNOOZE

2 drops Lavender essential oil
2 drops Vetiver essential oil
2 drops Sweet Marjoram essential oil

SWEET DREAMS

2 drops Lavender essential oil
2 drops Roman Chamomile essential oil
2 drops Sweet Marjoram essential oil

DREAM VIBES

3 drops Vetiver essential oil
3 drops Lavender essential oil
2 drops Frankincense essential oil

SLEEPY THYME

1 drop Sweet Orange essential oil
1 drop Thyme essential oil
1 drop Sweet Marjoram essential oil

PERSONAL INHALERS

Essential oil inhalers are an excellent way to enjoy the perks of essential oils even when you're not at home or unable to use a diffuser. They're portable, practical, and discreet. This blending and recipe guide will show you how to make your inhaler blends.

What You Will Need:

- Inhaler apparatus
- Label
- Essential oils for the blend you choose
- Fractionated coconut oil (optional)
- Tiny bowl
- Pipette
- Tweezers
- Surgical/Exam gloves

Plastic inhalers are typically made of four parts: a cover, a wick, a wick enclosure, and a cap. Aluminum inhalers are generally made of a glass vial, a wick, an aluminum screw-on top with air holes, an outer aluminum enclosure, and an aluminum cap.

Many other aromatherapy diffuser blends can be used as inspiration for creating inhaler blends. However, thoroughly research the safety precautions for each essential oil you plan to use in your blend and limit the number of drops to no more than 15 drops per inhaler.

WHAT TO DO FOR PLASTIC INHALER ASSEMBLY:

1. Mix the essential oils for your chosen blend in a tiny bowl.
2. If you do not want the inhaler to be intensely aromatic, add approximately 5-15 drops of fractionated coconut oil into your essential oil blend to weaken the scent. You will need to experiment with the dilution to achieve your desired aromatic strength.
3. Place the wick in the bowl.
4. Using your tweezers, rotate the wick around to absorb the essential oil blend completely.
5. Once the wick is saturated with the oil, use the tweezers to pick it up and place it in the wick enclosure (the part with a hole at the top).
6. Secure the end cap or butt onto the wick enclosure.
7. Screw the outer cover onto the wick enclosure.
8. Label your inhaler.
9. Keep the lid/cover on the inhaler when you are not using it.

FOR ALUMINUM ENCASED GLASS VIAL:

Follow steps 1-5, then continue with the following steps:

6. Place the wick inside the glass vial, leaving a small portion of the wick sticking out of the glass vial. Depending on the size of the wick, you may need to use your fingers to push it into the glass vial opening (wear surgical gloves).

7. Screw the metal piece with the inhaler holes onto the glass vial. Place the glass vial into the long, outer aluminum enclosure.

8. Slide the aluminum cap onto the top of the inhaler.

HOW TO USE YOUR ESSENTIAL OIL INHALER

- Remove the cap from your essential oil inhaler.
- Raise it to one nostril, ensuring that the tip of the inhaler does not come into direct contact with your nose (or other skin).
- Inhale as deeply as is comfortable.
- Repeat with the other nostril.
- Close the cap.
- If you experience any adverse reactions, discontinue using your inhaler immediately.

Check the safety information to ensure the oil is appropriate for personal use. Essential oil blends suggested in this book are for use by healthy adults with no serious underlying medical issues.

Cut the number of drops in half for children under six years of age. Inhaler blends are not recommended for children under three.

INHALER BLEND RECIPES

SLEEP TIGHT

5 drops Cedarwood essential oil
5 drops Lavender essential oil
5 drops Vetiver essential oil

DEEP DIVE

5 drops Patchouli essential oil
5 drops Sandalwood essential oil
5 drops Sweet Orange essential oil

RISE AND SHINE

5 drops Neroli essential oil
5 drops Petitgrain essential oil
5 drops Sweet Orange essential oil

BEDTIME STORIES

5 drops Lemon essential oil
5 drops Ylang Ylang essential oil
5 drops Cedarwood essential oil

BEDDY BYE TIME

5 drops Lavender essential oil
5 drops Roman Chamomile essential oil
5 drops Geranium essential oil

"DON'T GIVE UP ON YOUR DREAMS SO SOON, SLEEP LONGER."

– ANONYMOUS

ROOM

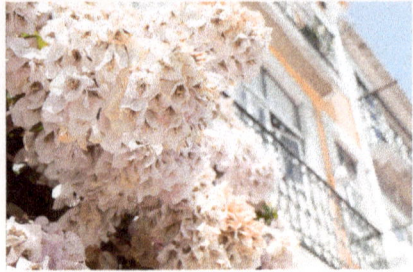

A room spray is a type of diffusion that quickly releases a concentrated amount of oil into the air. You will use approximately 30-40 drops of essential oil in hydrosol or mineral water and vodka if hydrosol is unavailable. Use as needed to create a special atmosphere.

SPRAY

To ensure the essential oils disperse throughout the hydrosol or another water-based carrier (and stay mixed), you will need to add a product called "Solubol," an all-natural dispersant. If you do not have this, you may substitute aloe vera or glycerin in its place.

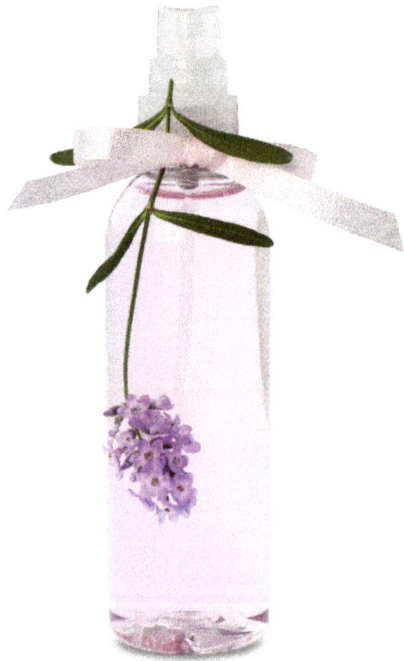

ROOM SPRAYS

Room sprays are great for changing the mood of a room. You may choose any fragrant hydrosol or floral water for your base. Some of the best ones for creating a pleasant, soothing atmosphere include Lavender and Roman Chamomile. If you want a more romantic feel for your space, you may wish to use Ylang Ylang or Neroli as your water-based carrier. Choose 2-3 oils to add to your blend. You can use the chart to determine which essential oils you would like to add to your blend.

What You Will Need:

- 18 - 24 drops top note essential oil
- 12 - 16 drops middle essential oil
- 6 - 8 drops base essential oil
- 2 oz (60 ml) PET plastic or glass spray bottle
- 1/2 teaspoon solubol or aloe vera gel
- glass bowl and stir rod
- funnel
- perfume strips
- 2 oz hydrosol, floral water, or distilled water

1. Remove the spray nozzle from the spray bottle – you will add your carrier and oils right into the spray bottle.
2. Choose three essential oils. Add the number of drops for each note. Check the scent when adding drops to make sure you are happy with the scent.
3. Replace the nozzle and cap and shake.
4. Create a nice label for your room spray.

ROOM SPRAY BLENDS

HIT THE SNOOZE

18 drops Mandarin essential oil
12 drops Neroli essential oil
6 drops Patchouli essential oil

SNORE NO MORE

18 drops Lemon Myrtle essential oil
12 drops Thyme essential oil
6 drops Vetiver essential oil

BEDDIE BYE

18 drops Sweet Orange essential oil
12 drops Clary Sage essential oil
6 drops Frankincense essential oil

SWEET DREAMS

18 drops Melissa essential oil
12 drops Marjoram essential oil
6 drops Sandalwood essential oil

DREAMLAND

18 drops Cilantro essential oil
12 drops Geranium essential oil
6 drops Rosewood essential oil

TIPS FOR A GOOD

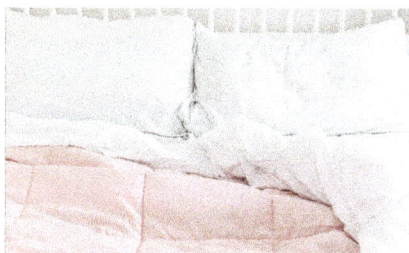

NIGHT'S SLEEP

Good sleeping habits (referred to as "sleep hygiene") can help you get a good night's sleep. It is important to take a step back and analyze your life to see if there are any issues causing anxiety or stress leading to insomnia. Tackling these problems can help to improve your sleep. Using essential oils and aromatherapy can help you relax, get ready for bed, and be better prepared for the next day.

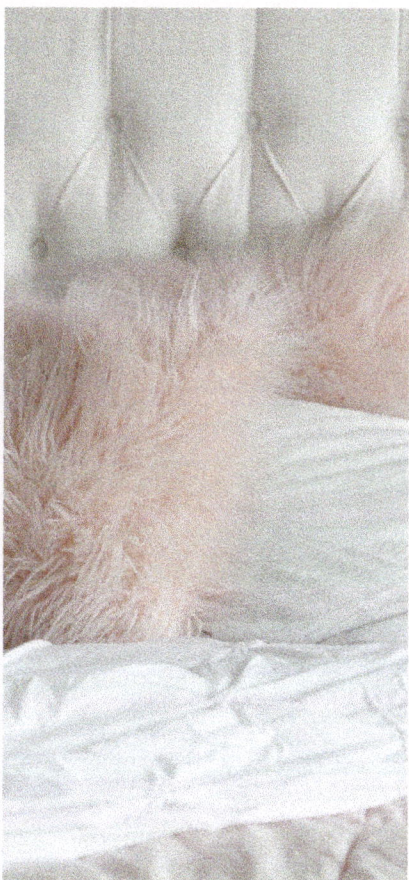

There are many ways you can improve your nighttime sleep ritual, such as taking a hot shower and sipping on warm tea before bed. Soothing, relaxing aromas, or a gentle aromatic massage can help you unwind after a long day. When it comes to sleep, consider your needs and use your favorite essential oil blends to help create a peaceful sleeping environment.

CREATE A CONSISTENT BEDTIME ROUTINE

You and your children can benefit from a routine with the same preparations every night before bed. This signals your body that it's time to start winding down and relaxing for sleep. It's okay if you can't follow the exact schedule every night. However, when you stick with it, you'll notice that both you and your youngsters respond well to the familiar steps leading up to a good night's rest.

CUP OF TEA

A way to calm down and prepare for sleep is to drink a cup of warm or hot tea before bed. Make sure your tea is not caffeinated, as stimulants can keep you awake. Add a drop or two of Bergamot or Roman Chamomile essential oil to your cup of tea for extra flavor and to help you relax before bed. For safety, ensure any oil you add to your tea has been approved for internal use and is safe for food and drinks.

SLEEPY SPACE

Your home should be a safe and restful place for your entire family. By making a few small changes, you can encourage healthy sleep habits for everyone.

CHILL OUT

Lowering the temperature in your home can help signal the body to prepare for bedtime. Even a couple of degrees can tell your body that you are finishing the day and getting ready for sleep.

UNPLUG

The adverse effects of using electronics for reading or entertainment right before bed include taking longer to fall asleep, less restful sleep, and increased tiredness upon waking. It's not worth sacrificing your rest, so turn off those devices! You may want to remove phones from the room.

PILLOW SPRAY

Invest in a comfortable pillow. Your pillow needs will differ depending on your sleeping habits (such as if you sleep on your side, back, or stomach). Another way to enjoy the benefits of essential oils is by applying them to your pillows and bedding to promote better sleep quality. Combine a few ounces of water and a few drops of essential oils in a spray bottle and spritz your pillows and bedding. When you lay down with your head on the pillows, you will be surrounded by essential oils' relaxing, comforting aroma.

USE A BEDTIME LINEN SPRAY ON YOUR SHEETS

Use a linen spray on all your linens to set the right tone for bedtime. Make a batch of linen spray to spray the linens and pillows. Parents of young children even spray this under the bed to help make them brave against the things that go bump in the night.

SOAK AWAY

Incorporating a lavender milk bath into your bedtime routine can be very beneficial. Lavender milk will nourish your skin while you relax and take time for yourself. Or, add a few drops of essential oils to a warm bath to help you calm down and comfort the body and mind before bed. Not only will a warm bath help soothe the body after a long day, but the essential oils will provide aromatic benefits to help you sleep better and wake fully rested. You can also add a few drops of oils to some Epsom salts and place them in the bottom of the bathtub. If you are a person who prefers showers to baths, you can use essential oils in the shower to help relax the mind and body before sleep. Sprinkle a few drops of a calming essential oil on the shower floor to allow the steam to disperse the aroma throughout the room. Remember to place the drops away from the path of the water so that your oils don't get washed down the drain right away.

SPLASH YOUR FACE WITH WATER

It's not just hygienic; it's scientific! Washing your face with cold water before bed can tell your body it's time to rest. Believe it or not, it's true.

JUST BREATHE

Try a simple breathing exercise the next time you have trouble falling asleep.

APPLY LOTION WITH OILS

For topical applications, add a few drops of a soothing essential oil to your body lotion and apply it to the body after showering. You will smell the aroma as you begin to wind down and sleep. Essential oils such as Clary Sage, Lavender, Roman Chamomile, and Ylang Ylang are calming oils that promote healthy sleep while nourishing the skin.

FUZZY SOCKS

Wear socks to bed to slumber more soundly. By doing so, your body is tricked into a more peaceful sleep. Therefore, adorn your feet with a pair of wonderfully soft, fuzzy socks for extra cuteness in bed.

CLEAR YOUR MIND

Sleep easily comes to those who can clear their minds of all worry. Anxiety can prevent you from thoroughly relaxing. Just let it go!

SLEEPY SONGS

Lullabies can help people of all ages relax and drift off to sleep. Choose a song without lyrics that is calming.

WHITE NOISE

If you're not fond of music, you could try white noise instead. Some people run a bathroom fan or vent to drown out street noise. Or, you could purchase a white noise machine that helps some drift off to sleep. Be careful not to make the white noise too loud, especially for babies.

LIGHTS OUT

Make sure your bedroom is quiet, dark, and relaxing. Shades or room-darkening curtains may help block streetlights.

SLEEPY HEAD

It's time for sleep. Your body is ready for bedtime. Now, clear your mind and focus on getting a good night's rest. Don't focus on anything at all.

AVOID LARGE MEALS

Never go to bed on a heavy meal. Its also advised to avoid caffeine and alcohol before bedtime.

EXERCISE

Get some exercise. Being physically active during the day can help you fall asleep more easily at night.

DIFFUSE

Turn on your essential oil diffuser while preparing for bed if it takes you a while to settle down for sleep. That way, you get the benefits of the calming aroma as you prepare to sleep, helping you relax quicker once you lie down. Use an oil diffuser with a timer to extend the aroma lingering in the bedroom while you sleep. This will help you sleep peacefully through the night.

AROMA NECK WRAP

Another great way to use essential oils is with a heating pad or neck wrap to warm and relax the body. It is easy to prepare and takes only a few minutes. You simply add a few drops of an essential oil to the outside fabric of a heating pad and place it around the neck or on the back for soothing warmth.

MOIST HEATING PAD

Here is an easy DIY non-electric heating pad that is perfect to use with essential oils. Moisten a small washcloth, then heat in the microwave until steamy. Place in a plastic Ziploc bag and open it slightly for the aroma to escape. Wrap a hand towel around it to retain the heat. Place it where you need it most, such as on the back of your neck or over your forehead. This method works well for children as well. Remember, some essential oils can be potent and must be diluted when used around children.

No more nights of tossing and turning. You'll be well on your way to sleep and enjoying the benefits of the oil fragrance long into the night. You now have essential oils' natural, potent power at your disposal. There will be no more counting sheep in your sleep routine. Incorporate these beneficial oils in your bedtime ritual and sleep, as you did as a child.

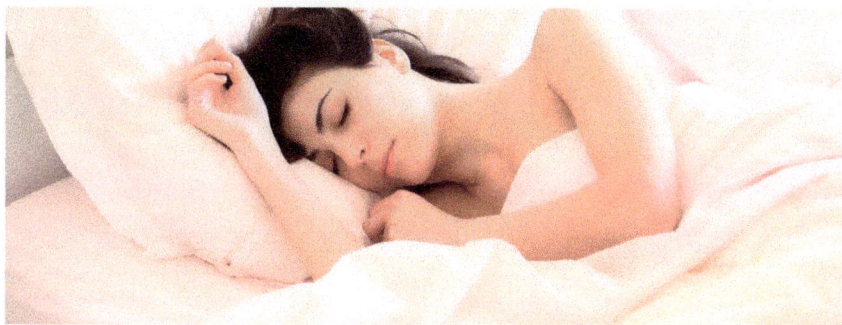

ESSENTIAL OIL SAFETY

In general, essential oils are safe for aromatherapy and therapeutic purposes. Nevertheless, safety must be exercised due to their potency and high concentration. Please read and follow these guidelines to obtain the maximum effectiveness and benefits.

Avoid sunbathing, tanning booths, or saunas immediately after applying essential oils topically.

Be careful to avoid getting essential oils in the eyes. If you splash a drop or two of essential oil in the eyes, use a small amount of olive oil (or another carrier oil) to dilute the essential oil and absorb it with a washcloth. If severe, seek medical attention immediately.

Take extra precautions when using oils with children. Never use undiluted essential oils on babies, and always store your essential oils out of the reach of children.

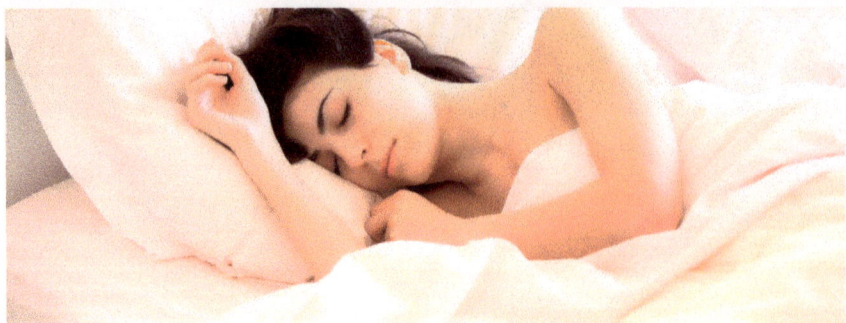

If a dangerous quantity of essential oil has been ingested, immediately drink olive oil and induce vomiting. The olive oil will help slow down its absorption and dilute the essential oil. Do not drink water—this will speed up the essential oil absorption.

Never use oils undiluted on your skin. Always dilute with a carrier oil. Stop using oil immediately if there is redness, burning, itching, or irritation. Be sure to wash your hands after handling pure, undiluted essential oils.

If you are pregnant, lactating, suffer from epilepsy, have cancer, liver damage, or another medical condition, use essential oils under the care and supervision of a qualified Aromatherapist or medical practitioner.

Less is best when taking essential oils internally. Take fewer drops every 4-6 hours versus more at one time.

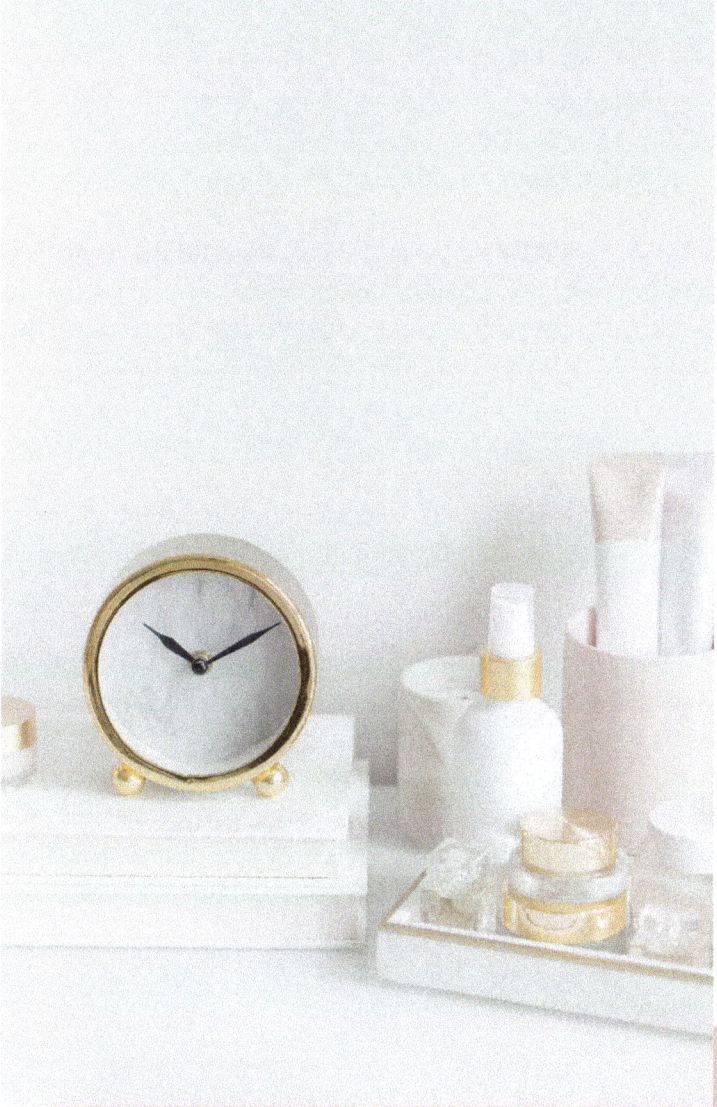

CHAPTER NINE

TOPICAL USE

Topical use is applying the essential oils directly to the skin's surface; always use a carrier for topical use. Ways to use essential oils topically include:

- Roller Bottle
- Lotion
- Massage Oil
- Bath Salts

You can apply the essential oil(s) of choice to the back of the neck, feet, legs, etc., mixed with a lotion or carrier oil. Try combining a couple of oils to create a synergistic blend for multiple health benefits.

When using an essential oil topically, dilute it with a carrier oil. Essential oils are potent and direct application, or "neat" may cause irritation to the skin. Also, combining essential oils with a carrier base oil such as almond or coconut oil can add additional benefits to your treatment.

Topically is one of the easiest and most effective ways to use essential oils. For example, massage stimulates blood circulation while reducing muscular tension, aches and pain, and inflammation. Also, it significantly reduces stress and can offer comfort and peace of mind, allowing you to sleep. Caution should be exercised when using topical aromatherapy preparations around drug injection sites or areas of the body where transdermal medications are in use (i.e., estrogen or nicotine patches, etc.).

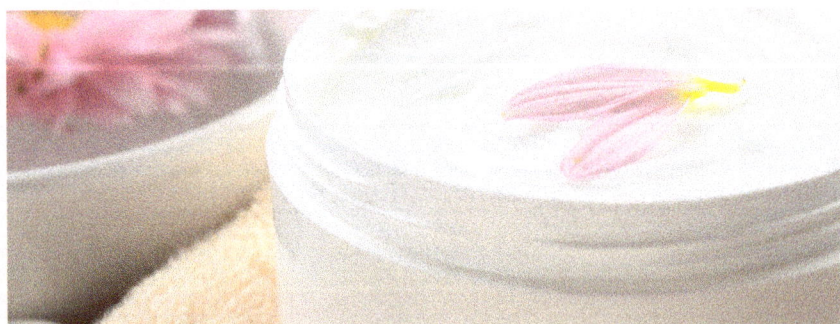

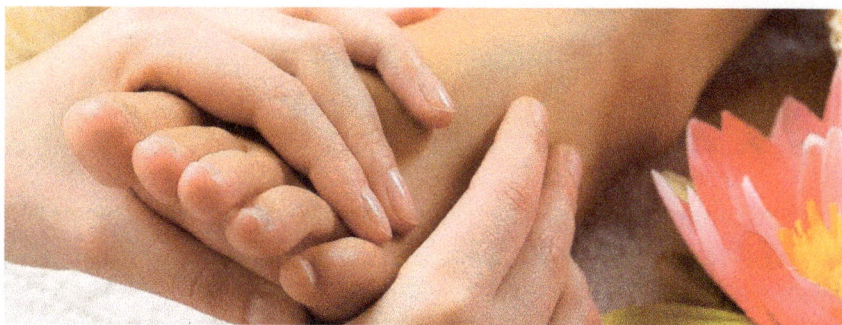

The absorption of certain essential oil chemical compounds has been confirmed through analysis of blood concentrations, with maximum levels attained in as little as 10 minutes.

WAYS TO USE ESSENTIAL OILS TOPICALLY

- **Roll-On** – Use a rollerball applicator to apply oil blend where needed. Reapply several times a day as needed.
- **Rub On** – Rub 1-2 drops of essential oil directly "neat" on the joint or affected area. Or rub an essential oil or essential oil blend on the bottom of your feet each evening before bed.
- **Massage** – Massage an essential oil blend (with a carrier oil) over the body for several minutes. Reapply as desired. Apply to the back of the neck, joints, and feet. Applying essential oils topically can be quite beneficial since the oils will permeate your skin due to their transdermal properties. Massage and therapeutic baths will be your best methods of treatment. They stimulate circulation, help eliminate toxins, and absorb the minerals needed to function correctly.
- **Bath** – Sea salt baths are great for relaxation because they stimulate circulation. Sea salts and Epsom salts are great to use in baths.

Massages stimulate circulation and help eliminate toxins.

BATH

For a full bath, mix 8-10 drops of essential oil into two ounces of sea salts or a cup of milk, then pour into a running bath. Agitate water in a figure-eight motion to make sure the oil is mixed well, preventing irritation to mucous membranes. Another method is to add essential oils after the bath has been drawn. Mix essential oils into a palm full of liquid soap, shampoo, or a tablespoon of Jojoba oil and swish around to dissolve in the tub. Soak for 15-20 minutes. Adding salts to the bath helps relax muscles which can help you to relax. Adding Lavender or Clary Sage essential oil to a carrier oil or under running bathwater will help induce sleep.

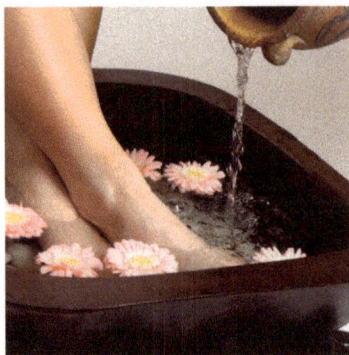

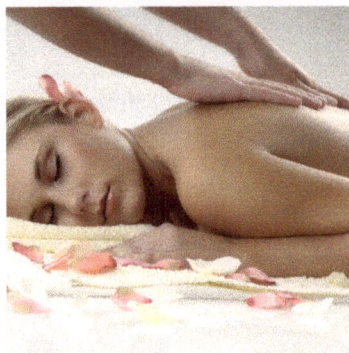

SHOWER

While showering, add a drop or two of essential oil to a washcloth with liquid soap or body wash and rub it on the body.

Several techniques used in massage therapy can incorporate the use of essential oils.

MASSAGE

A variety of techniques used in massage therapy can incorporate the use of essential oils. Add 6-9 drops of essential

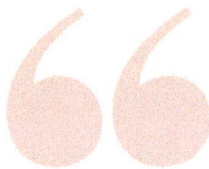

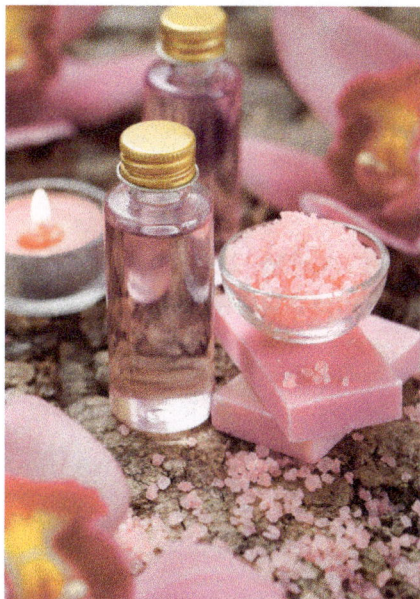

oil to 1 tablespoon of your favorite carrier oil to massage into the body.

LOTIONS/CREAMS

Blending essential oils in an unscented, natural lotion/cream base allows you to benefit from the therapeutic qualities of the essential oil, giving you a non-oily way to apply essential oils. This is especially useful for someone with a skin condition that does not do well with oils. The dilution rate for using essential oils in a lotion base is no more than 2%. For adults, use 20 drops of essential oil to four ounces of lotion. For children and the elderly, use ten drops of essential oil to four ounces of lotion.

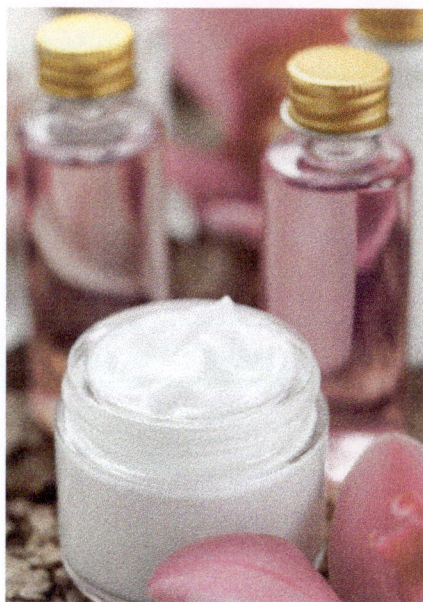

BODY OILS

Mix 30 drops of essential oil per ounce of cold-pressed carrier oil such as coconut oil. Choose an all-purpose oil that relieves stress, tension, and headaches and smells terrific.

MASSAGE OIL

Essential oils have been used for many years to enhance relaxation during a massage. Using an essential oil with a calming, relaxing property as part of a relaxing massage is a great way to promote a good night of sleep.

To apply, warm a few drops of essential oil with a teaspoon of a favorite carrier oil in your hand, rub between the palms, and then massage the oil into the temples or neck muscles. Massaging these two areas with essential oils is an effective way to calm and relax you before bedtime.

This can also be applied to the shoulders, arms, back, legs, or feet to help relax these areas. Diluting essential oils with carrier oil will help the oils be absorbed into the skin and linger while you drift off to sleep. Please make sure the essential oil you choose is safe for topical use. Some oils are potent and irritate the skin if not recommended for topical use.

As a general rule of thumb: Use two to three drops of essential oil per teaspoon of carrier oil (follow individual recipes when available). A full-body massage takes about one to two ounces of carrier oil. Any natural carrier oil (except mineral oil) is okay to use when preparing a massage blend. As a general rule, add 10-12 drops of essential oil to 30ml carrier oil. For children and the elderly, use only 5-6 drops of essential oil to 30ml of carrier oil.

Keep In Mind When Choosing Your Carrier Oil:

- **Odor:** A few carrier oils have a distinct odor. When added to an essential oil, it may alter the aroma.
- **Absorption:** Your skin can absorb some carrier oils better than others.
- **Skin Type:** Depending on your skin type, some oils may irritate or worsen a skin condition such as acne.
- **Shelf Life:** Some carrier oils can be stored for longer periods than others without going bad.

CHAPTER TEN

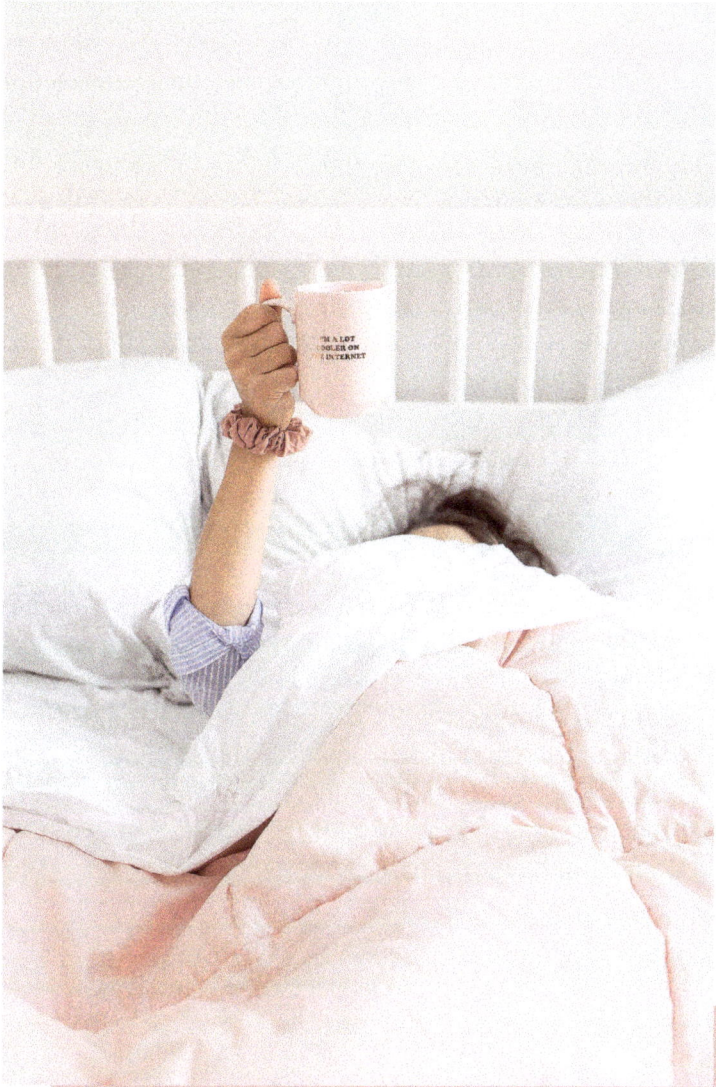

ORAL USE

Certain essential oils can be taken internally for relaxation. Check labels carefully to ensure the essential oils you choose are safe for ingestion. Not all essential oils are safe for taking orally.

If you are considering ingesting essential oils, you will want to treat your essential oils like powerful medicines because that is what they are. Taking an oil orally is nearly ten times stronger than when applied topically, so starting with a tiny amount and increasing gradually is wise. While many essential oils are safe when used internally, some are not. Be sure to read about the oil and do your research to know any warnings or contradictions. Also, you will want to be aware of proper dosage protocols. The necessary internal dose and frequency depend on age, size, and health condition, varying from person to person.

One essential oil company stated on their website, "The recommended internal dose of essential oils is 1–5 drops, depending on the oil or blend." Taking more than that is not advantageous; in fact, it can be harmful. It is better to take a smaller dose, which can be repeated every 4–6 hours as needed. A low daily dose is recommended for extended internal use.

Ingestion of certain essential oils may not serve to be the most efficient method for absorption into the bloodstream. They are absorbed into systemic circulation via the digestive tract. However, essential oils may lose some active principal compounds when taken orally due to the first-pass hepatic metabolism.

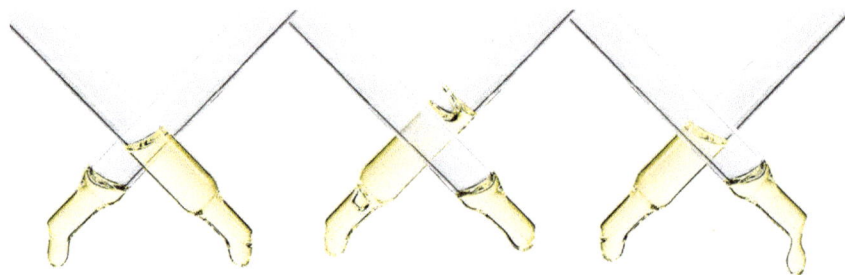

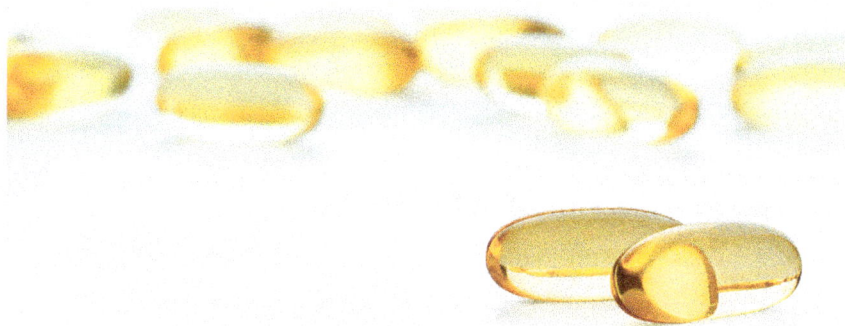

There are several methods for taking essential oils. In this book, internal use will comprise consuming essential oils by mouth in a vegetable capsule, adding oil to honey, or on a sugar cube. Essential oils taken by mouth, not in a capsule, may be absorbed through the cheeks, tongue, or throat lining. Essential oils are highly concentrated and potent—treat like you would with any other highly concentrated pharmaceutical. When using essential oils internally, it is recommended to seek the advice of a certified medical practitioner who is also trained in aromatherapy or a Clinical Certified Aromatherapist who is also trained in internal ingestion for the best protocol.

Essential oils are highly concentrated and potent – treat like you would with any other highly concentrated pharmaceutical.

When using essential oils internally, doses in the range of one to three drops, one to two times a day (for adults), follow a protocol appropriate for your health. Caution should be used as all essential oils are not recommended for ingestion. You should receive guidance from a qualified health professional before ingesting essential oils. Please store your oils in a safe place away from children. Using the appropriate amount of essential oil in a vegetable capsule that has been properly diluted can be maximally absorbed by the gut for the whole-body effect. But like medicines, essential oil ingestion carries the potential for side effects, mild to severe, including seizures and poisoning.

- **Capsules** – Add one or two drops of essential oil to a "00" gelatin capsule filled with a carrier oil such as olive or fractionated coconut oil to buffer the essential oil. Take orally as you would with traditional supplements. A single oil or essential oil blend may be used in this way. For example, a capsule is filled with 20% essential oil diluted with 80% vegetable oil (one ml=20 drops approximately). Each "00" capsule holds approximately 0.7-.91ml or 14 drops, and "0" capsules hold ten drops of oil. Enteric-Coated Gelatin Capsules could also be used since they do not release the essential oil until they are in the small intestine.
- **Juice or Water** – Add one or two drops of essential oil to a small glass of juice. Stir to blend well, as oil will tend to float on the surface. A solubol can be added as a dispersant to distribute the oils.
- **Tea** – Add one or two drops of essential oil to a teaspoon of

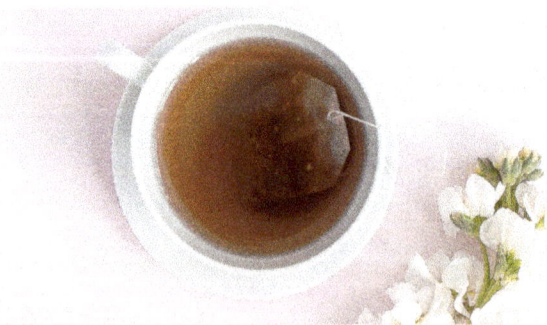

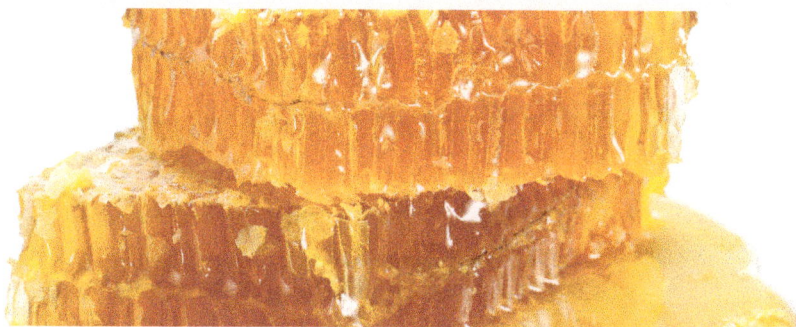

honey and stir into a cup of tea or warm water. Be sure not to overheat the water, as oils will evaporate. Sip slowly.

- **Swishing** – Add several drops of essential oil to a cup of water and swish around the mouth before swallowing.
- **Sugar Cube** – Use a dropper to add one or two drops of essential oil to a cube of sugar. It can be taken directly or added to a drink.
- **Honey** – Essential oils can be blended with honey water. Mix 1-2 drops of essential oil into 1 Tsp. honey, add warm water, and drink. Or add 1-2 drops of essential oil or oil blend to a tablespoon of honey, stir with a toothpick, and take orally.

The recommended oral dosage with essential oils for adults is 1-3 drops, two to three times a day. The maximum daily dose is 12 drops. Some essential oil websites recommend up to 20 drops a day, which is relatively high and is therefore not recommended. Some professionals recommend using essential oils two weeks out of the month or taking one drop three times a day for an extended period. Others suggest using 1-2 drops, two to three times a day for five days, and taking two days rest. Either way, taking breaks in your essential oil usage is advisable.

INGESTION METHOD

WHY TAKE ESSENTIAL OILS BY MOUTH?

It is widely believed that essential oils are suitable for anxiety, sleeplessness, and other related conditions. Essential oils safe for internal use can be absorbed through the mucous membranes (nose, under the tongue, and the throat lining). The oral route ushers essential oils into the digestive tract, readily absorbing them into the bloodstream. Some of the issues that respond to this method include:

- Relaxation
- Insomnia
- Anxiety

MEDIUMS FOR INTERNAL USE

Some of the following mediums may be used for the oral route: sugar cube, honey, gelatin capsules, bread, rice flour capsules, dried powdered herb capsules, herbal tinctures, neutral tablets, milk, fatty oil capsules, charcoal, tinctures, alcohol, and syrups.

GELATIN CAPSULES

Gel capsules with fractionated coconut or olive oil are an optimum way to ingest harsh essential oils such as cinnamon or thyme. Such oils can be used for certain nervous system imbalances such as stress, insomnia, and anxiety.

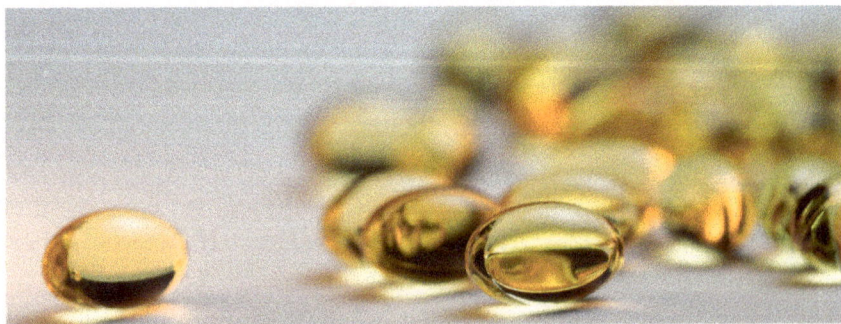

NEUTRAL TABLET

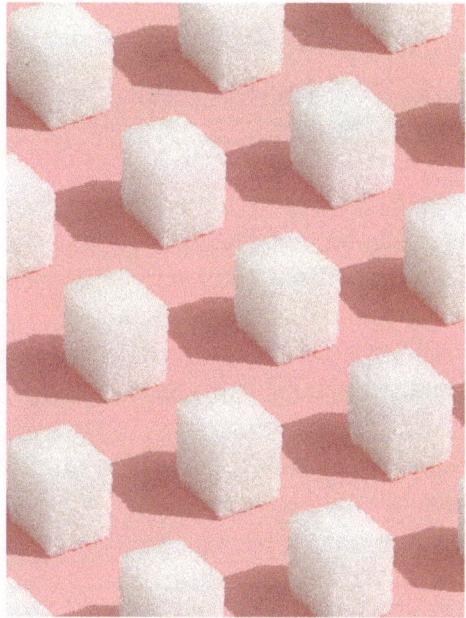

Neutral tablets are another widely used excipient for essential oils. They dissolve quickly and are absorbed in the mucosa of the mouth. For safety, ensure the tablet has completely absorbed the essential oils before swallowing it. You can swallow the tablet once it has dried.

Other alternatives include sugar cubes, bread, charcoal, rice flour capsules, syrups, and dried powdered herb capsules.

NEUTRAL TABLETS ARE ANOTHER POPULAR METHOD FOR SAFELY INGESTING ESSENTIAL OILS.

MIXING ESSENTIAL OILS IN WATER

To emulsify the essential oils in the water, two products help make them more soluble: Solubol and Dispera. These are recommended to reduce throat irritation and digestive issues.

Solubol is a natural, non-alcoholic dispersant that quickly disperses essential oils into the water. Blend one part of essential oil with four parts of Solubol. Shake well. Add 3-4 drops to a glass of water or juice. This is also an excellent way to use essential oils in the bath.

Dispera is similar to Solubol but contains 70% alcohol solution. Dispera also aids the absorption of essential oils by the digestive tract. Combine 80-90% Dispera to 20-10% essential oil and place one to two drops in a glass of water.

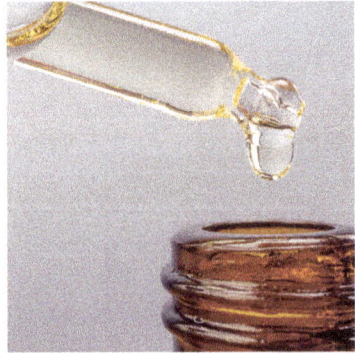

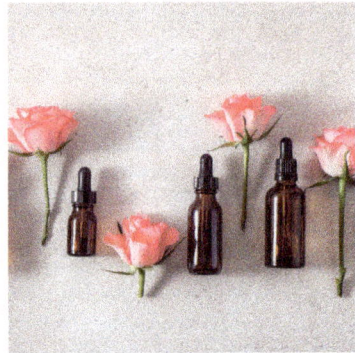

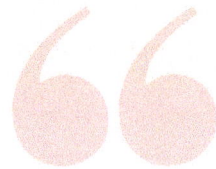

> *To emulsify the essential oils in the water, two products help make them more soluble: Solubol and Dispera.*

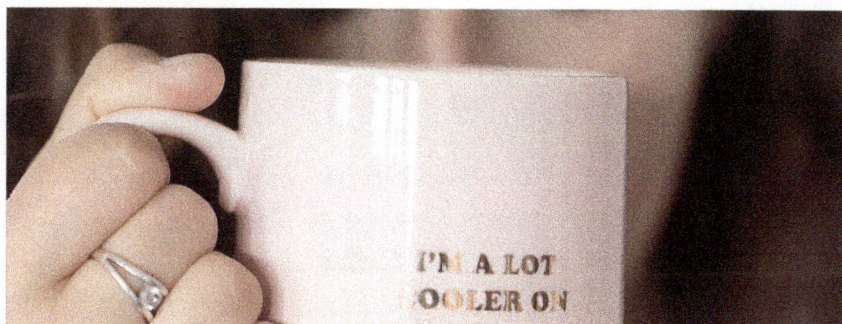

WHEN SHOULD YOU TAKE ESSENTIAL OILS INTERNALLY?

Essential oils should typically be taken before a meal. Another option, especially when taking strong combinations (like thyme and cinnamon), is to take it halfway through a meal to not upset or irritate the stomach lining.

THE SUBLINGUAL ROUTE

The word 'sublingual' refers to applications placed under the tongue. Essential oils are administered by placing one drop of essential oil under the tongue or by placing one or two drops on a neutral tablet and placing the tablet under the tongue to dissolve.

This method speeds the absorption of the molecules into the bloodstream and avoids the effect of hepatic first-pass metabolism and the gastrointestinal tract. It is most readily absorbed in this manner.

The reticulated vein underneath the tongue absorbs the essential oil components. It then transports them from the tiny facial veins to the larger jugular and brachiocephalic veins.

ADVANTAGES OF SUBLINGUAL DOSING:

- Fast acting (peak levels reached in 10-15minutes)
- Easy to self-administer
- Bypasses extensive hepatic first–pass metabolic process
- Sublingual dosing does not require swallowing, which is suitable for patients with Dysphagia
- The absorption rate is 3 to 10 times greater than through the oral route

WHEN TO USE THE SUBLINGUAL ROUTE AND DOSAGE

The sublingual route is recommended for acute insomnia or acute anxiety.

DOSAGE

Sublingual dosage: 6 drops of essential per day maximum for adults with 1 to 3 drops per dose of non-irritating essential oils.

For adults: 1-2 drops 3-4 times/day
For adolescents: 2 drops 2 times/day
For children over seven years old: 1 drop two times/day

When taking sublingual drops, it is recommended to use an eye dropper and bring it in front of a mirror to be sure the application gets under the tongue. You may also use it on a neutral tablet as well.

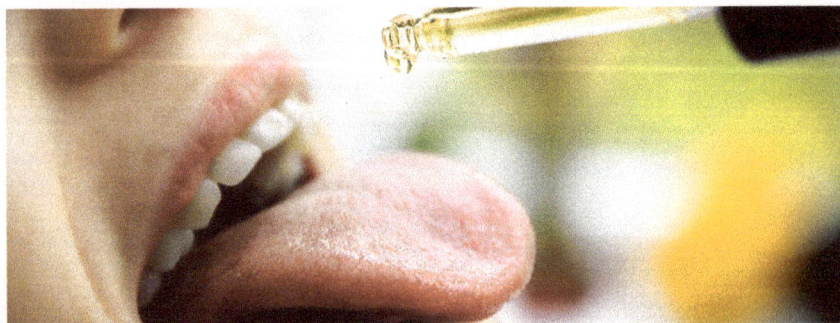

Buccal dosage: for mouth conditions, place one drop of essential oil in the mouth between the upper and lower gums and cheek area. This can also be placed on neutral tablets.

When to use: The best time to take sublingual essential oils is before eating a meal.

WHICH ESSENTIAL OILS SHOULD YOU USE FOR SUBLINGUAL USE?

You should use only non-irritating essential oils such as Lavender, Coriander, Lemon, etc. The only downside to this is possibly an unpleasant taste based on the flavor of the oils.

HOW LONG SHOULD I USE ESSENTIAL OILS?

It is recommended to continue essential oil therapy for a few days or more following relief of symptoms to ensure complete healing occurs. A general rule of thumb in aromatherapy is that for every year you have suffered from a chronic condition, it could take one month of therapy to correct the condition. For acute conditions, if you do not obtain results within an hour or so, try a different essential oil or method of application. Everyone responds differently, and you may need to use more or less essential oil, depending on how your body reacts.

BUILDING UP A TOLERANCE TO ESSENTIAL OILS

It is safe to use the recipes in this book as recommended several times a day for a week or more. However, it is recommended to limit the use of the same oil or essential oil blend to twenty-one days and then take a week break. Rotating your blends and using different oils or blends is also recommended.

ROTATE YOUR OILS

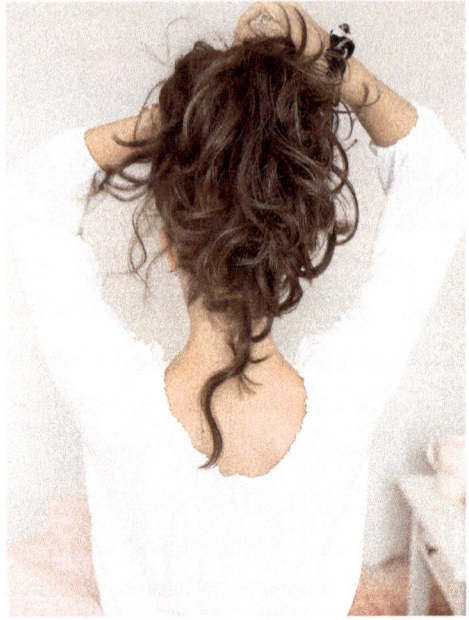

After regularly continued use of the same oil or blend, you should rotate your blends and use different oils. This is recommended for two reasons. First, this reduces the possibility of a risk of sensitization to the essential oil or blend that you are using.

Secondly, this also reduces the chance of your body developing resistance or becoming acclimated to the effectiveness of the essential oils you are using. In other words, the essential oil blend may no longer work or provide the same positive benefits it once did.

ALWAYS ROTATE YOUR BLENDS AND USE DIFFERENT OILS.

CHAPTER ELEVEN

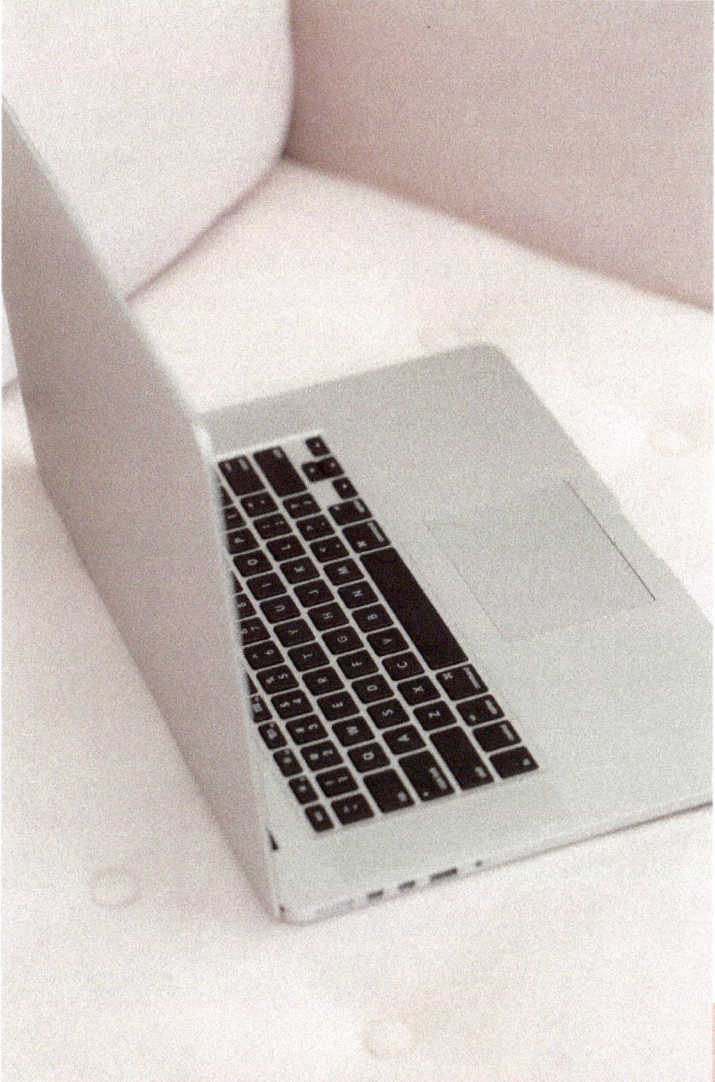

CARRIER OILS

When you use essential oils topically, you will want to dilute them with a carrier or vegetable oil. Carrier and infused oils are used to dilute essential oils and absolutes by offering the necessary lubrication and moisture to the skin for aromatherapy.

Carrier oils come from nuts, seeds, or kernels that contain essential fatty acids, fat-soluble vitamins, minerals, and other crucial nutrients. You will find a variety of carrier oils to choose from, each possessing different therapeutic properties.

Distinct from essential oils, carrier oils do not contain aromatic scents (or only a very faint scent) and evaporate due to their large molecular structure. For this reason, most consider carrier oils just a vehicle for applying essential oils to the skin in massage. However, they offer healing properties that essential oils do not possess. Your aromatherapy experience can be significantly enhanced by choosing the best combination of carrier and essential oils.

SHELF LIFE OF CARRIER OILS

A carrier oil's shelf life, the length of time before a particular oil begins to turn rancid, can be significantly influenced by heat and light. You will want to store your oils in a cool, dark place to preserve their freshness and, in some cases, refrigerate, as heat and sunlight can shorten their shelf life. When refrigerating, oils may appear cloudy but will regain their transparent state upon returning to room temperature. If you have a large amount of carrier oil on hand, you can freeze the unused portion until ready for use.

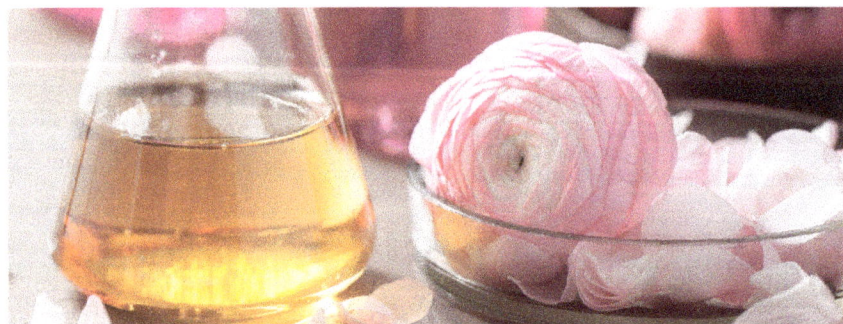

Carrier Oil	Shelf Life
Almond (sweet)	12 months
Apricot Kernel	6-12 months
Argan	24 months
Avocado	12 months
Borage	6 months
Carrot Seed	12 months
Cocoa Butter	3-5 years
Coconut (fractionated)	Indefinite
Coconut (virgin)	2-4 years
Evening Primrose	6-12 months
Grapeseed	3-6 months
Hemp Seed	12 months
Jojoba	Indefinite
Olive	12-18 months
Safflower	24 months
Shea Butter	Indefinite
Walnut	12 months

When carrier oils are used with essential oils topically, they provide a mechanism for the volatile oils to be transported more effectively. Most essential oils, when applied externally, move through the body system in an hour. A carrier oil, thicker than a volatile oil, "holds" the essential oil in place, delivering longer-lasting healing.

Essential oils in aromatherapy are highly concentrated and potent. Although there are only a few exceptions to using essential oils 'neat' or undiluted (such as Lavender and Chamomile), it is ideal always to use a carrier oil with your essential oils to avoid having an adverse effect or skin irritation.

TIP: A massage oil blend with 10-15% essential oil and 85-90% carrier oil will ensure a powerful massage oil that is smooth and great-smelling.

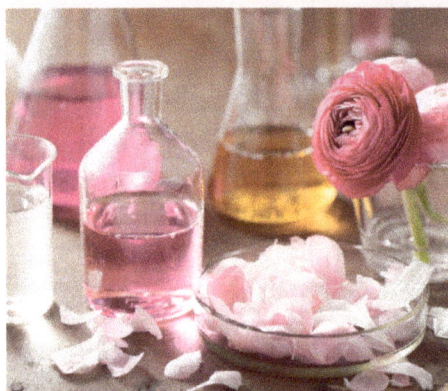

Carrier oils provide the much-needed lubrication, allowing hands to move freely over the skin, and helping with the absorption of essential oils into the body. Choose a carrier oil that is light, non-sticky, and that can effectively penetrate the skin. Always check the label to ensure it's 100% pure, unrefined, and cold-pressed.

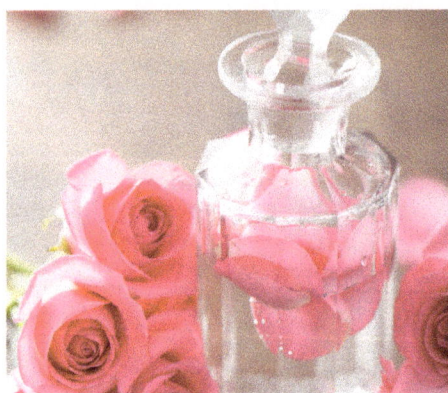

TIP: Try not to mix too much of your favorite massage blend in advance if you don't plan on using it right away.

With the vast selection of carrier oils, each with various therapeutic benefits, choosing one will depend on the area it's being applied to, the treatment plan, and any skin sensitivities. When using oil for massage, viscosity is an important consideration. Some carrier oils may work better than others in specific applications. For example, Grapeseed oil is generally very thin while Olive oil is much thicker, and others such as Sunflower and Sweet Almond have viscosities halfway between these extremes. You can easily blend carrier oils to combine their properties of viscosity, absorption rate, and benefits.

TIP: When shopping for a good quality carrier oil, make sure it's cold-pressed to retain all its natural qualities.

Almond Oil is one of the most useful, practical, and moderately priced carrier oils. It is ideal for all skin types as it moisturizes and reconditions the skin with its satiny smooth texture. This pale-yellow oil quickly absorbs into the skin, leaving your skin feeling soft and non-greasy. Sweet Almond relieves itching, soreness, dryness, and inflammation and is especially beneficial for eczema. As a lightly nutty refined oil rich in fatty acids, proteins, and Vitamin D, it is everyone's favorite massage base oil for loosening stiff muscles and achy joints.

Dilution: Can be used at 100%.

Coconut Oil (Fractionated) seems to be quickly becoming the carrier oil of choice because of its broad use in alternative medicine and healing. While it is fractionated, no change has been made chemically. Instead, its molecular structure 'fraction' has been separated, allowing it to remain liquid at room temperature, making it much more helpful in aromatherapy. Coconut oil is perfect as a moisturizer for the body while delivering its many health benefits. Its light, easily absorbable texture gives skin a smooth satin effect with virtually no scent of its own and indefinite shelf life.

Dilution: Can be used at 100%.

Coconut Oil (Virgin) has an incredible balance of natural saturated fatty acids with antibacterial and antiviral properties not found in other oils. Coconut oil is perfect as a skin conditioner for nearly all skin conditions and is believed to stimulate hair growth. It has a light, aromatic coconut scent that becomes solid at room temperature. For this reason, blending with other carrier oils in your body care products is recommended. It is fully digestible and is considered a healthy cooking oil. Several virgin coconut oils are high in antioxidants which are positively associated with reducing oxidative stress and thus lowering blood pressure.

Dilution: It can be used alone directly, but it is recommended to use 10-25% dilution with other carrier oils.

Grapeseed Oil is a lovely, light green, and odorless oil, useful as a base oil for many creams, lotions, and carrier oil. Grapeseed oil is pressed from the seeds of a grape and contains OPCs, flavonoids, vitamin E, resveratrol, and fatty acids. It is non-allergenic and has very high levels of linoleic acid, with traces of proanthocyanidins, which are very potent antioxidants. It is especially beneficial for all skin types because of its natural non-allergenic properties. Grapeseed works well, especially when other oils do not absorb well, without leaving a greasy feeling after application. Grapeseed makes an ideal carrier oil for body massage bases. Saturation takes longer than some other carrier oils.

Dilution: Can be used at 100%.

Jojoba Oil is bright and golden in color and is known as one of the best oils (actually a liquid wax) for hair and skin. It penetrates the skin quickly and is excellent for nourishing and healing inflamed skin, psoriasis, eczema, or dermatitis. It is suitable for all skin types and promotes a healthy, glowing complexion by gently unclogging the pores and lifting embedded impurities. Jojoba is suitable for all aromatherapy uses other than a full-body massage. And, because of the oil's antioxidants, it does not become rancid and can even prevent rancidity in other oils.

Dilution: It can be used at 100%, but many use a 10% dilution with other carrier oils due to its price.

Olive Oil (Extra Virgin) is light to medium green in color, with a slightly dense texture. It is very soothing and carries disinfecting and healing properties. Olive oil is legendary since it has been used over the centuries for multiple purposes, but due to its overpowering scent, this oil does not work well for massages. However, it is beneficial in some lotions for burns or scars. Olive is very helpful for dry, damaged, or split hair and is soothing for inflamed skin such as eczema. The "virgin" indicates it comes from the first pressing of the fruit. The "extra" means it comes from a single source. Extra virgin olive oil is beneficial for high blood pressure because it contains more vitamin E than virgin, pure or extra light varieties.

Dilution: Can be used at 100% or 25-50% dilution with another carrier oil blend.

Shea Butter is a thick, lustrous butter (not a carrier oil) with excellent therapeutic properties. It contains powerful anti-inflammatory properties known to reduce swelling and pain. Shea butter leaves the skin feeling smooth and healthy and combats many skin conditions. Shea butter has a very cream-like consistency, so you may want to warm and blend with other carrier oils for a thinner or liquid consistency if desired.

Dilution: Can be used at 100% or diluted at 25-25% with another carrier oil for blending purposes.

TIP: Mineral oil and petroleum jelly should never be used as a carrier oil in therapeutic blending. These are derivatives of petroleum production from gasoline and are not of natural botanical origins. It prevents toxins from escaping the body through perspiration and is believed to also prevent the body from adequately absorbing vitamins and utilizing them, including essential oil absorption.

DILUTION RATE FOR YOUR BLENDS

When creating an essential oil blend for sleep, you will need to consider the amount of carrier oil to use for dilution. Be sure to dilute correctly to make sure your blend is safe to use and doesn't waste your precious essential oil.

The following dilution rate chart shows you the amount of pure therapeutic essential oil to use with your carrier oil. Use a measuring spoon to add the carrier oil and a dropper to add your essential oils.

Most essential oils should be diluted for topical applications, using a 1-3% concentration of essential oils (in some cases, 5-10%). This means 6-24 drops of essential oil will be used per ounce of carrier. Therapeutic massage blends will contain between 1%-5% essential oils.

For example, adding two to three drops of pure essential oil will need diluting by adding about a teaspoon of carrier oil. For children or senior citizens, cut this amount in half.

SIMPLE EVERYDAY DILUTION CHART

Essential Oil	To	Carrier Oil
1 drop		¼ teaspoon
2-5 drops		1 teaspoon
4-10 drops		2 teaspoons
6-15 drops		1 Tablespoon
8-20 drops		4 teaspoons
12-30 drops		2 Tablespoons

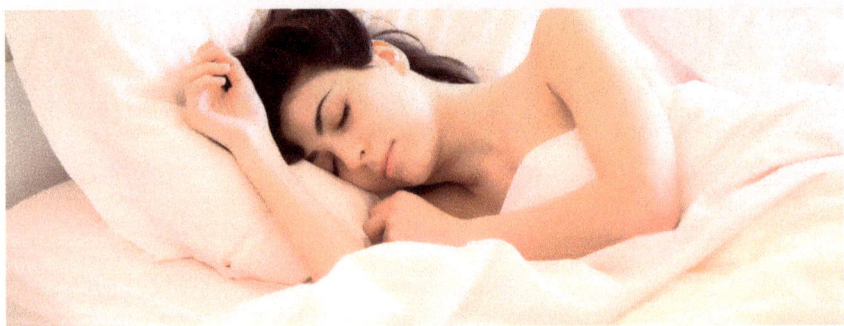

EQUIPMENT USED FOR CREATING BLENDS FOR SLEEP

Before getting started, you will want to gather your supplies, such as bottles, droppers, and containers.

Glass Bottles, preferably dark, in 5ml, 10ml, and 15ml sizes with orifice reducers (plastic dropper), can be used to make topical essential oil blends.

Glass Spray Bottles are great for making room sprays, facial spritzers, or cleaning solutions. You will find these in sizes of 1-ounce, 2-ounce, 4-ounce, 8-ounce, and 16-ounce.

Small Glass Tubs are perfect for bath salts, facial creams, salves, scrubs, or other bath blends. These come in various shapes and sizes, from 2-ounce to 8-ounce.

Pocket Diffusers are perfect as "personal inhalers" to carry in a pocket or purse with your favorite blend. They come with a cotton wick that saturates the essential oil inside the chamber. These are terrific for taking to work or school!

You will need waterproof labels for your bottles and want them in all shapes and sizes.

CREATING BLENDS FOR SLEEP

Coming up with your essential oil blend for insomnia is easy to do when you follow the blend by note technique. Your essential oil blend will contain one or more oils from each of the above categories: Base note, Middle note, and Top note (see chart). Some apothecaries recommend using a fourth note, a fixative, or bridge notes such as Lavender, Chamomile, Marjoram, or Myrrh. The bridge is what helps the other three oils meld.

Some oils made fall into more than one category. This is possible because of the many components essential oils possess and the synergy effect a blend might draw out of that oil. However, make this work to your advantage when creating your therapeutic blends. For instance, there may come a time when you have several middle note essential oils on hand to choose from but no top notes for your condition. In this case, you could use an essential oil that may be a top note and middle note as your top note and choose a different oil as your middle note. Follow this guide when orchestrating your blends, and let your nose have the final say.

Often Vitamin E oil is used for topical blends. The following chart contains essential oils known to be beneficial for sleep. Each essential oil is listed by its common name and note classification: Top, Middle, and Base.

OILS FOR SLEEP CHART

TOP	MIDDLE	BASE
Bergamot	Roman Chamomile	Cedarwood
Cilantro	German Chamomile	Frankincense
Lemon	Clary Sage	Jasmine
Lemongrass	Cypress	Opoponax
Lemon Myrtle	Dill	Patchouli
Mandarin	Lavender	Rose
May Chang	Lavandin	Rosewood
Melissa	Linaloe Berry	Sandalwood
Neroli	Marjoram	Spikenard
Petitgrain	Rosalina	Valerian
	Rose	Vetiver
	Geranium	Violet Leaf
		Ylang Ylang

Top Notes are oils that have a light, fresh aroma. It is the first scent you smell after applying a blend to the skin. Although they quickly evaporate, the top note is what gives us our first impression of a blend. Familiar top notes include Lemon, Bergamot, Orange, Lime, and other citrus oils. Most top notes are made up chemically of aldehydes and esters, which are generally found in oils from fruits, flowers, and leaves.

For Therapeutic Blending: Use 3 to 15 drops of a top note per 30 ml (or one ounce) carrier.

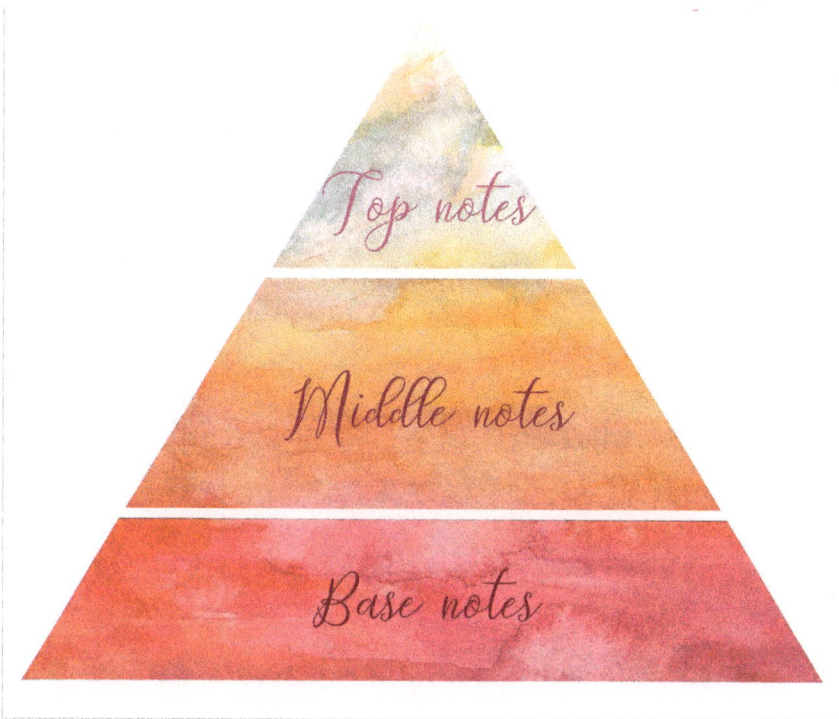

Middle Notes, also referred to as heart notes, are usually the inspiration for an aromatic blend and include floral scents such as Roman Chamomile, Lavender, or Neroli. It is generally considered the heart of the blend as it often covers any unpleasant odors that may come from the base notes. Essential oils classified as middle notes are sometimes referred to as enhancers, equalizers, or balancers. Chemically, these are monoterpene alcohols found mostly in herbs and leaves. Examples of essential oil middle notes include Lavender, Roman Chamomile, Cypress, Geranium, Juniper Berry, Rosemary, and Peppermint. Middle notes are what we smell when the scent from the top notes fades. This scent often evaporates after 15 seconds. The middle note can last 2-4 hours in the body, and the "heart" of the blend can play on the emotions. Middle notes are often found in flowers, leaves, and needles. They also bring together the top and base note as a "synergy" in a blend.

For Therapeutic Blending: Use 2 to 10 drops of a middle note per 30 ml (or one ounce) carrier.

Base Notes, usually the backbone and foundation of the blend, are what the users will remember most about a particular fragrance. The scent of base notes will last the longest in the air and are what you smell after about 30 seconds of applying it to your skin. The base note is added to the mixture first. Examples of essential oil base notes include Vanilla, Sandalwood, Patchouli, Frankincense, Cinnamon, or other earthy and woodsy scents. Typically, a therapeutic blend has only one base note oil as it will stay the longest on the skin and can last up to 72 hours in the body. Aromatic blends can have one or more base oils to add character. Chemically speaking, base notes are made up of sesquiterpenes or diterpenes and are mainly found in roots, gums, and resins. Though therapeutic blends typically contain one base note while aromatic blends may contain more than one, for any blend to be successful, it must have a combination of all three notes.

For Therapeutic Blending: Use 1 to 5 drops of a base note per 30 ml (or one ounce) carrier.

When making an essential oil blend for your sleep blend, mix the extracts in order, starting with the base note, then the middle note, and finally, the top note. This ensures your blend will create an aroma known as a "bouquet" by staying in tune with odor intensity and finding notes that strike a chord and harmonize well together in therapeutic properties. Remember, for every base note drop, you add two drops of the middle note and three drops of the top note. This will ensure that your blend is well-rounded, has all three notes, and is chemically balanced between monoterpenes, sesquiterpenes, and phenols.

Tip: Everyone is unique, and what works for your condition may not work well for another. Be willing to try different combinations to find which oils help you the most.

MAKING YOUR FIRST SLEEP BLEND

Now that you have learned how many drops of each note to use in your essential oil blend and have checked the precautions, it's time to start blending.

1. Gather all the necessary equipment: bottles, pipettes, essential oils, paper towels, labels, vials, and containers.
2. Ensure the counter space is clean, and the area you work in is well-ventilated. You may want to put down wax paper (or a paper towel) to prevent any damage to the countertop from accidental spills. This will also make cleaning up much more manageable.
3. If you are using essential oils that are new to you, place one drop of the oil on a test strip (or small piece of paper) and wave it under your nose. Inhale the fragrance. If this fragrance is not what you had in mind, choose another oil and test again. You will want to do this with each oil until you have settled on the ones you want to use for your blend. It is a good idea to have a can of coffee grounds to smell after each fragrance to clear your palette.
4. Once you have chosen the three oils for your blend, wave all three test strips fanned out beneath your nose and see if you like them. Remember that if you despise the scent, you may hesitate to use it regularly.
5. Check the safety precautions for the essential oils you have chosen to ensure there aren't any contradictions. Always consider any other health conditions, such as epilepsy or medications that may cause an adverse effect. The safety precautions must always be considered for the method you choose in their usage and for the person you are formulating the blend for.
6. Choose a new, clean bottle to use. Using a pipette, extract each essential oil into the bulb to place in your bottle. You may need to squeeze more than once to get the desired amount. Remember to use a separate pipette or glass eye dropper for each oil used. Add your base note essential oil first, one drop at a time. This is typically the most

viscous or thickest oil. Next, add the middle note essential oil, followed by the top note essential oil. Use only the exact number of drops your recipe calls for. One drop of too many can alter the results. Replace the cap on the bottle and shake to mix oils.

7. Add your essential oil blend to a carrier oil (lotion, gel, sea salts, etc.) and blend well to distribute the oils. What you use as your carrier and how much to add will depend on which application method (Massage Blend, Bath Blend, Room Spray, etc.) you choose.

TIP: Always leave ½ inch of headspace at the top of your bottle allowing your pure essential oil blend to breathe and expand.

CHAPTER TWELVE

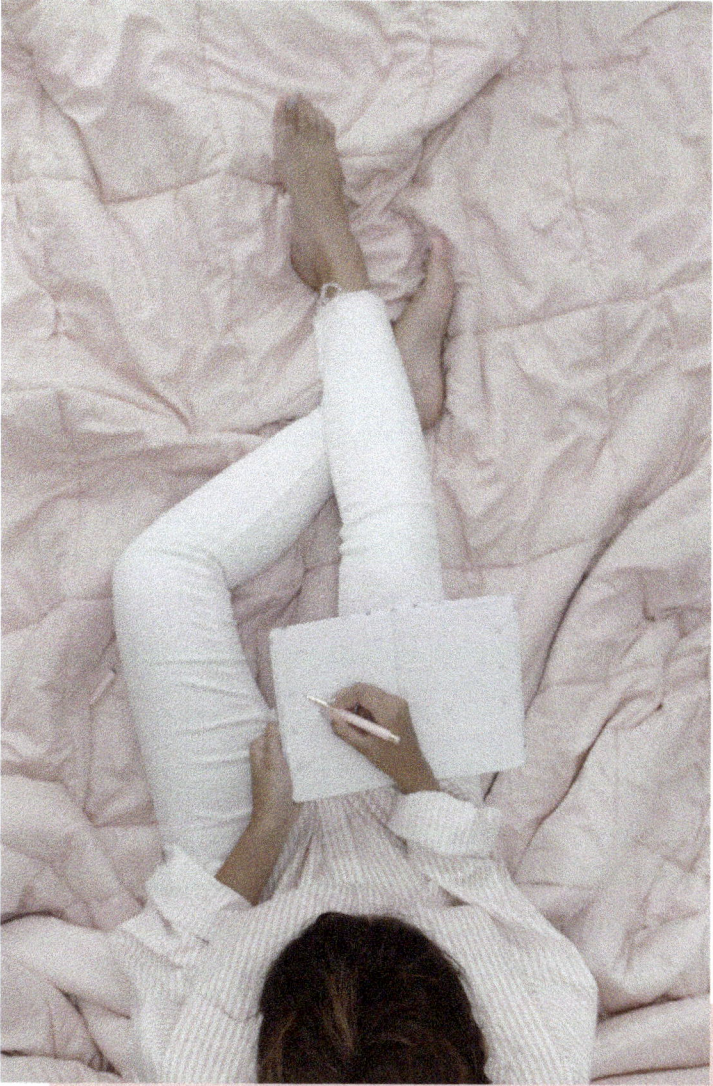

RECIPES

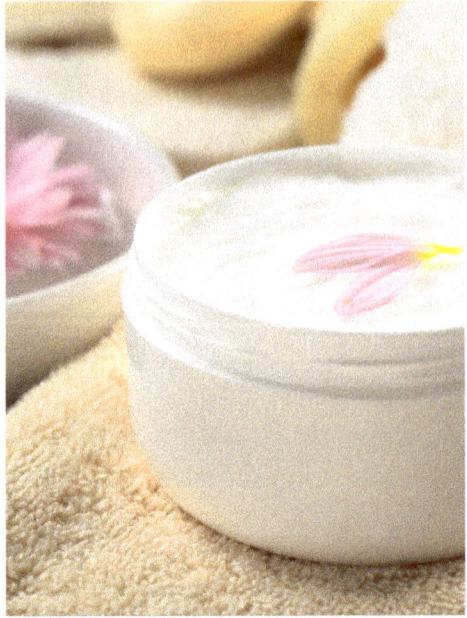

In this chapter, you will find various recipes for relaxation and sleep. Since there are so many reasons for insomnia, you will want to try different combinations of oils to improve efficacy. Results will vary from person to person. You may also want to come up with your sleep blend based on the oils you have on hand.

TRY DIFFERENT COMBINATIONS OF OILS TO IMPROVE THEIR EFFECTIVENESS.

DIY SLEEP MASSAGE OIL

Massage oil for feet and legs to help induce sleep.

WHAT YOU WILL NEED:

4-6 drops Lavender essential oil
4-6 drops Vetiver essential oil
4-6 drops Lemon essential oil
1 tablespoon Fractionated Coconut oil (or another favorite carrier oil)
15 ml Glass Bottle

WHAT TO DO:

1. In a clean bottle, add the essential oils, then fill with the carrier oil, such as fractionated coconut oil or grapeseed oil.
2. Replace cap and shake to blend.
3. Apply as needed after showering or before bed.

DREAM DROPS ROLL-ON BLEND

Sleep like a baby tonight after rolling on these relaxing oils.

WHAT YOU WILL NEED:

5 drops Lavender essential oil
5 drops Vetiver essential oil
5 drops Frankincense essential oil
5 drops Ylang ylang essential oil
5 drops Bergamot essential oil
2 teaspoons Fractionated Coconut oil
10 ml Roller bottle

WHAT TO DO:

1. Remove the cap and roller ball, then add your essential oils.
2. Fill the remaining space with Fractionated Coconut oil.
3. Replace roller ball and cap. Shake to mix.
4. Use as needed by applying to the legs and feet before bed.

KNOCK OUT ROLL-ON BLEND

This blend will knock you down for the countdown.

WHAT YOU WILL NEED:

3 drops Patchouli essential oil
2 drops Sweet Orange essential oil
2 drops Frankincense essential oil
2 teaspoons Fractionated Coconut oil
10 ml Roller bottle

WHAT TO DO:

1. Remove the cap and roller ball, then add your essential oils.
2. Fill the remaining space with Fractionated Coconut oil.
3. Replace roller ball and cap. Shake to mix.
4. Use as needed by applying to the soles of the feet before bed.

SLEEPY TIME BATH BLEND

Add this essential oil blend to a warm bath before retiring.

WHAT YOU WILL NEED:

12 drops Bergamot essential oil
8 drops Lavender essential oil
4 drops Cedarwood essential oil
3 drops Valerian essential oil
2 drops Roman Chamomile essential oil
½ cup Epsom Salts
Small Tub or Container

WHAT TO DO:

1. Place Epsom salts in a small container. Add oils into the salts and stir.
2. Pour salt mixture into the running bath water and swish around to blend.
3. Soak and enjoy before bedtime.

DEEP SLEEP BATH BLEND

Add this essential oil blend to a steamy bath before sleep.

WHAT YOU WILL NEED:

2 drops Lavender essential oil
2 drops Valerian essential oil
2 drops Roman Chamomile essential oil
½ cup Dead Sea Salts
Small Tub or Container

WHAT TO DO:

1. Place the Dead Sea salts in a small tub or container. Add oils into the salts and stir.
2. Pour salt mixture into the running bath water and swish around to blend.
3. Soak and enjoy before bedtime.

SLEEP TIME BATH OIL BLEND

Add this essential oil blend to a hot bath before retiring to bed.

WHAT YOU WILL NEED:

3 drops Roman Chamomile essential oil
2 drops Bergamot essential oil
2 drops Frankincense essential oil
½ cup Himlayan Salts
Small Tub or Container

WHAT TO DO:

1. Place the Himalayan salts in a small tub or container. Add oils into the salts and stir.
2. Pour salt mixture into the running bath water and swish around to blend.
3. Soak and enjoy before bedtime.

SNORE NO MORE MASSAGE BLEND

Massage oil onto throat, chest and back of neck to stop snoring.

WHAT YOU WILL NEED:

6 drops Marjoram essential oil
4 drops Geranium essential oil
4 drops Lavender essential oil
2 drops Eucalyptus essential oil
2 drops Cedarwood essential oil
1 tablespoon Fractionated Coconut oil (or another favorite carrier oil)
15 ml Glass Bottle

WHAT TO DO:

1. In a clean bottle, add the essential oils, then fill with the carrier oil, such as fractionated coconut oil or jojoba oil.
2. Replace cap and shake to blend.
3. Apply as needed to throat, chest, and back of neck before bed.

SWEET DREAMS ROOM SPRAY

Mist room generously with this lovely spray and sleep soundly.

WHAT YOU WILL NEED:

4 drops Lavender essential oil
2 drops Cedarwood essential oil
2 drops Sweet Orange essential oil
1 drop Ylang Ylang essential oil
1-ounce Lavender Hydrosol or Mineral Water
1-ounce Glass Spray Bottle

WHAT TO DO:

1. In a clean spray bottle, add the essential oils, then fill with a hydrosol or mineral water.
2. Replace spray nozzle and shake to blend.
3. Spray generously in the bedroom and on bed linens before retiring.

SPA DREAMS ROOM SPRAY

Mist room generously with this invigorating spray and be refreshed.

WHAT YOU WILL NEED:

3 drops Lavender essential oil
4 drops Lime essential oil
2 drops Peppermint essential oil
1-ounce Lavender Hydrosol or Mineral Water
1-ounce Glass Spray Bottle

WHAT TO DO:

1. In a clean spray bottle, add the essential oils, then fill with a hydrosol or floral water. You can also substitute with mineral water.
2. Replace spray nozzle and shake to blend.
3. Spray generously in the bedroom and on bed linens before retiring.

BEDTIME ROOM SPRAY

Spray this refreshing room spray to prepare your mind for a relaxing atmosphere.

WHAT YOU WILL NEED:

5 drops Roman Chamomile essential oil
5 drops Clary Sage essential oil
5 drops Bergamot essential oil
1-ounce Hydrosol or Mineral Water
1-ounce Glass Spray Bottle

WHAT TO DO:

1. In a clean spray bottle, add the essential oils, then fill with a hydrosol or floral water. You can also substitute with mineral water.
2. Replace spray nozzle and shake to blend.
3. Spray generously in the bedroom and on bed linens before retiring.

SLEEP IN ROOM SPRAY

Spritz your bed linens and throughout the room generously before retiring.

WHAT YOU WILL NEED:

5 drops Vetiver essential oil
4 drops Patchouli essential oil
6 drops Mandarin essential oil
1-ounce Mineral Water
1-ounce Glass Spray Bottle

WHAT TO DO:

1. In a clean spray bottle, add the essential oils, then fill with mineral water. You can also substitute with floral water.
2. Replace spray nozzle and shake to blend.
3. Spray generously in the bedroom and on bed linens before retiring.

BEDROOM SPRITZER

Spritz your bed pillows and sheets generously before retiring.

WHAT YOU WILL NEED:

5 drops Lavender essential oil
4 drops Petitgrain essential oil
6 drops Mandarin essential oil
1-ounce Hydrosol or Floral Water
1-ounce Glass Spray Bottle

WHAT TO DO:

1. In a clean spray bottle, add the essential oils, then fill with hydrosol or floral water. You can also substitute with mineral water.
2. Replace spray nozzle and shake to blend.
3. Spray generously in the bedroom, on pillows and sheets before sleep.

ROMANTIC LINEN SPRAY
Spritz your bed pillows and sheets for a romantic evening.

WHAT YOU WILL NEED:

15 drops Sandalwood essential oil
15 drops Neroli essential oil
2 drops Rose essential oil
2 drops Jasmine essential oil
4 ounces Hydrosol or Floral Water (your choice)
4-ounce Glass Spray Bottle
Solubol (such as Polysorbate 20; follow the directions for usage)

WHAT TO DO:
1. In a clean spray bottle, add the essential oils, then fill with hydrosol or floral water. You can also substitute with mineral water.
2. Replace spray nozzle and shake to blend.
3. Spray generously in the bedroom, on pillows and sheets before sleep.

MUSCLE RELAXER MASSAGE OIL
Let this blend work its magic when insomnia is caused due to overworked stiff muscles.

WHAT YOU WILL NEED:

1 drop Rosemary essential oil
3 drops Eucalyptus essential oil
2 drops Lavender essential oil
1 teaspoon Fractionated Coconut oil (or another favorite carrier oil)
15 ml Glass Bottle

WHAT TO DO:
1. In a clean bottle, add the essential oils, then fill with the carrier oil, such as fractionated coconut oil or jojoba oil.
2. Replace cap and shake to blend.
3. Massage this blend into your affected tight muscle area.

RESTLESS LEG MUSCLE BLEND

This is a great option for you if you often don't get enough sleep because your muscles tend to tighten up and you can't seem to relax.

WHAT YOU WILL NEED:

4 drops Lavender essential oil
2 drops Sweet Marjoram essential oil
2 drops Roman Chamomile essential oil
2 drops Bergamot essential oil
1 drop Ylang Ylang essential oil
1 drop Valerian Root essential oil
Fractionated Coconut oil
10 ml Glass Roller Bottle

WHAT TO DO:

1. Add essential oils together in a glass bottle.
2. Fill the remaining space with fractionated coconut oil.
3. Replace ball insert and cap. Shake well to mix.
4. Use this blend as needed throughout the day and evening before bed to relieve muscle tension.
5. To apply, massage it into the muscles of the legs and bottom of your feet. Use as needed.

PEACE BE STILL ROLLER BLEND

This blend works best for insomnia caused by anxiety. Let the sweet essence of this essential oil blend quiet your mind and spirit.

WHAT YOU WILL NEED:

2 drops Roman Chamomile essential oil
2 drops Sweet Marjoram essential oil
2 drops Lavender essential oil
10 ml Fractionated Coconut oil (or another carrier oil)
1 ml Glass Roller Bottle

WHAT TO DO:

1. In a glass roller bottle, add essential oils.
2. Fill the remaining space with your carrier oil.
3. To use, roll this blend over the neck, back of head, and temples.
4. To use as a diffuser blend, omit the carrier oil and add to your diffuser before bed.

STRESS HEADACHE ROLLER BLEND

When insomnia is caused by stress or a headache that won't quit.

WHAT YOU WILL NEED:

2 drops Sweet Orange essential oil
2 drops Lavender essential oil
2 drops Geranium essential oil
10 ml Fractionated Coconut Oil (or another carrier oil)
10 ml Glass Roller Bottle

WHAT TO DO:

1. In a clean bottle, add the essential oils, then fill with the carrier oil, such as fractionated coconut oil or jojoba oil.
2. Replace roller and cap and shake to blend.
3. Massage this blend into the temples and back of the head.

MOMMA'S LITTLE HELPER MASSAGE OIL

This sleep aid will help you get the rest you need.

WHAT YOU WILL NEED:

5 drops Lavender essential oil
5 drops Frankincense essential oil
5 drops Cedarwood essential oil
5 drops Bergamot essential oil
1 tablespoon Fractionated Coconut Oil (or another carrier oil)
15 ml Glass Bottle

WHAT TO DO:

1. Combine all oils into a small, dark-colored bottle.
2. Cap the bottle tightly, and shake well to blend.
3. Take a small amount into your hand and rub gently over the body before retiring.
4. If you prefer, the carrier oil can be omitted and the blend can be used in a diffuser instead.

ELEPHANT DREAMS BLEND

This blend should be made in advance for those times when you feel nauseous.

WHAT YOU WILL NEED:

2 drops Sweet Orange essential oil
2 drops Peppermint essential oil
2 drops Mandarin essential oil
1 tablespoon Fractionated Coconut Oil (or another carrier oil)
15 ml Glass Bottle

WHAT TO DO:

1. Combine all oils into a small, dark-colored bottle.
2. Cap the bottle tightly, and shake well to blend.
3. Take a small amount into your hand and rub gently over your stomach.
4. If you prefer, the carrier oil can be omitted and the blend used in a diffuser instead.

SUPER SNOOZE BATH OIL BLEND

After soaking in a warm bath apply this bath oil as a delightful treat. This one will ensure a better night's sleep.

WHAT YOU WILL NEED:

3 drops Lavender essential oil
2 drops Roman Chamomile essential oil
1 drop Ylang Ylang essential oil
1 drop Clary Sage essential oil
1 drop Sweet Marjoram essential oil
1 ounce Almond or Coconut oil
Small Glass Bottle or Container

WHAT TO DO:

1. Pour the carrier oil through a funnel into the corked container, leaving about an inch at the top.
2. Add essential oils to the container. Stir well to mix.
3. Replace cap and agitate the bottle gently.
4. Let it sit for 2-3 days before using.
5. For use, pour ½ – 1 teaspoon into the palm of your hand and gently massage into the body after a bath.

SWEET SLUMBER BATH OIL BLEND

Add this essential oil blend to a relaxing bath before retiring.

WHAT YOU WILL NEED:

3 drops Bergamot essential oil
2 drops Cedarwood essential oil
2 drops Sweet Marjoram essential oil
½ cup Himlayan Salts
Small Tub or Container

WHAT TO DO:

1. Place the Himalayan salts in a small tub or container. Add oils into the salts and stir.
2. Pour salt mixture into the running bath water and swish around to blend.
3. Soak and enjoy before bedtime.

BASIC BATH SALTS BLEND RECIPE

You can use Dead Sea, Himalayan, or Epsom salts for this basic bath salts recipe. Soak in a bath with this incredible blend to soothe the day's stress. Your bath salts can be made in advance and stored in a pretty container for convenience.

WHAT YOU WILL NEED:

2 cups Epsom Salts
1 cup Sea Salts
1 cup Baking Soda
30 drops Top Note essential oil
20 drops Middle Note essential oil
10 drops Base Note essential oil
Wide Mouth Jar or Container

WHAT TO DO:

1. Add essential oils together in a container. Stir to mix.
2. Add sea salts and mix well to saturate the salts with the oils thoroughly.
3. Add bath salts and swish in the tub to mix thoroughly in a running bath.

Tip: Check precautions for oils that may cause skin sensitivity. It is not recommended for children.

BASIC BATH OIL BLEND RECIPE

After a long day, soaking in a warm bath with a relaxing essential oil blend can be a delightful treat. Not only does it help take the edge off tense muscles, but it also ensures a better night's sleep.

WHAT YOU WILL NEED:

1 cup Almond oil or Coconut oil
30 drops Top Note essential oil
20 drops Middle Note essential oil
10 drops Base Note essential oil
Corked container
Crystal beads, dried flowers, tiny seashells, etc. (Optional)

WHAT TO DO:

1. Pour the carrier oil through a funnel into the corked container, leaving about an inch at the top.
2. Add essential oils to the container. Stir well to mix.
3. Cork the container and agitate the bottle gently.
4. Let it sit for 2-3 days before using. Add decor to your bottle.
5. For use, pour ½ – 1 teaspoon into the palm of your hand and gently massage into the body after a bath.

BASIC NASAL INHALER BLEND RECIPE

Filling a new nasal inhaler with your essential oil blend is an effective way to experience the therapeutic power of essential oils when suffering from sleeplessness. Inhalers are also great to use for anxiety and restlessness. They are small enough to carry in a pocket or purse and have on hand for immediate relief. Add 15-18 drops of your essential oil blend to your inhaler.

WHAT YOU WILL NEED:

9 drops Top Note essential oil
6 drops Middle Note essential oil
3 drops Base Note essential oil
Glass Dropper
Small Plastic Inhaler

WHAT TO DO:

1. In a container, mix essential oils. Stir well to mix.
2. Use a glass or disposal dropper to fill the nasal inhaler.
3. Carry and take a whiff as needed.

BASIC FOOT OIL BLEND RECIPE

A luxurious foot treatment with essential oils can readily deliver healing throughout the body. The sensitive skin and tissues of the feet take a lot of abuse and deserve a special blend that can easily be massaged in.

WHAT YOU WILL NEED:

1 ounce (30ml) Almond oil
3 drops Top Note essential oil
2 drops Middle Note essential oil
1 drop Base Note essential oil
1-ounce Glass Bottle

WHAT TO DO:

1. In a container, mix essential oils. Stir well to combine.
2. Add carrier oil to the bottle, replace the lid and shake to blend.
3. Massage oil blend into feet after a bath or shower or before bed. Wear soft, cotton socks to bed.

BASIC CAPSULE BLEND RECIPE

Here is a simple recipe for making an essential oil capsule for sleep. It is one of the best ways to take essential oils internally and bypass unpleasant tastes. You can use 1-2 drops of essential oil per capsule (depending on size).

WHAT YOU WILL NEED:

1-2 drops Essential Oil* (20%)
Carrier Oil (80%)

WHAT TO DO:

1. Separate the two parts of the capsule. Remove the top half (wider cap). You will only be filling the bottom half.
2. Add essential oil directly into the capsule, one drop at a time, using a glass dropper. This needs to be done carefully, not to add too many drops or drip oil on the side of the capsule, which will make it sticky.
3. Fill the remaining space with olive, coconut, pomegranate, etc.
4. Take the capsule immediately after filling it. These capsules will begin to dissolve right after filling them.
5. Take one capsule once in the morning and once in the evening, or as prescribed by your healthcare provider.

*ONLY USE ESSENTIAL OILS THAT ARE SAFE TO INGEST.

BASIC ROLL-ON OIL BLEND RECIPE

This basic recipe can be used to create a roll-on bottle applicator for your essential oil blend, depending on the oils you have on hand. Keep track of what you add or change, so you'll know how to make your favorite blends later.

WHAT YOU WILL NEED:

½ ounce Jojoba oil
9 drops Top Note essential oil
6 drops Middle Note essential oil
3 drops Base Note essential oil
Glass Roller Bottle

WHAT TO DO:

1. Add your carrier oil, such as Jojoba, to a dark container.
2. When adding essential oils, start with the base note and then add the middle note, followed by the top note. As you add each one, check the scent to ensure it is what you want.
3. Insert the ball and apply 2-3 times a day.

BASIC BODY LOTION BLEND RECIPE

Do you want to try a good body lotion recipe? Why not make your own by following these simple instructions?

WHAT YOU WILL NEED:

4 ounces Unscented Lotion, Hydrosol, or carrier oil
18 drops Top Note essential oil
12 drops Middle Note essential oil
6 drops Base Note essential oil
Glass Bottle or container

WHAT TO DO:

1. Add carrier oil to the container.
2. Add essential oils starting with your base note essential oil first, then the middle note, and finally the top note essential oil.
3. Recap and shake well to mix.
4. Use two to three times a day.

OTHER BOOKS

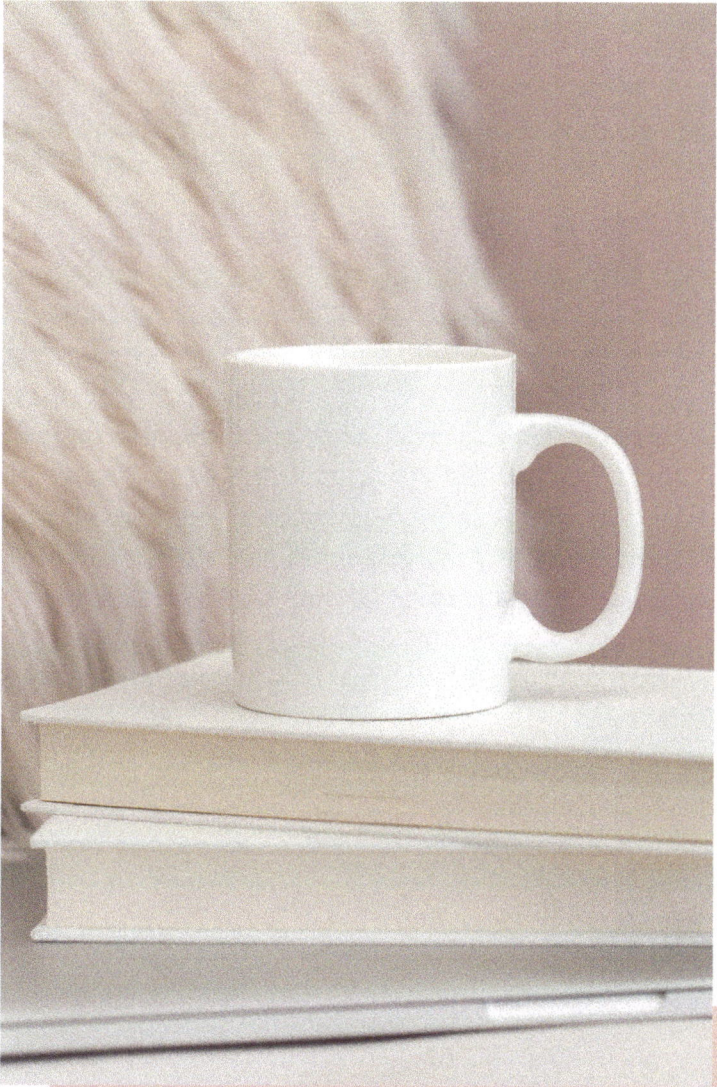

OTHER BOOKS BY REBECCA PARK TOTILO

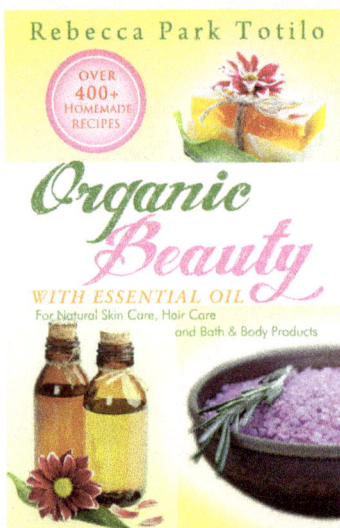

Organic Beauty With Essential Oil: Over 400+ Homemade Recipes for Natural Skin Care, Hair Care and Bath & Body Products

Sweep aside all those harmful chemically-based cosmetics and make your own organic bath and body products at home with the magic of potent essential oils! In this book, you'll find a luxurious array of over 400 eco-friendly recipes that call for breathtaking fragrances and soothing, rich organic ingredients satisfying you head to toe. Included you'll find helpful tips you can have the confidence knowing which essential oil to use and how much when creating your own body scrub, lip butter, or lotion bar! Discover how easy it is to make bath treats like fragrant shower gels, dreamy bubble baths, luscious creams and lotions, deep cleansing masks and facials for literally pennies using essential oils and ingredients from your kitchen.

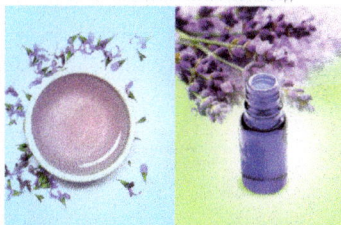

Heal With Essential Oil: Nature's Medicine Cabinet

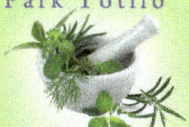

Using essential oils drawn from nature's own medicine cabinet of flowers, trees, seeds and roots, man can tap into God's healing power to heal oneself from almost any pain. Find relief from many conditions and rejuvenate the body. With over 125 recipes, this practical guide will walk you through in the most easy-to-understand form how to treat common ailments with your essential oils for everyday living. Filled with practical advice on therapeutic blending of oils and safety, a directory of the most effective oils for common ailments and easy to follow remedies chart, and prescriptive blends for aches, pains and sicknesses.

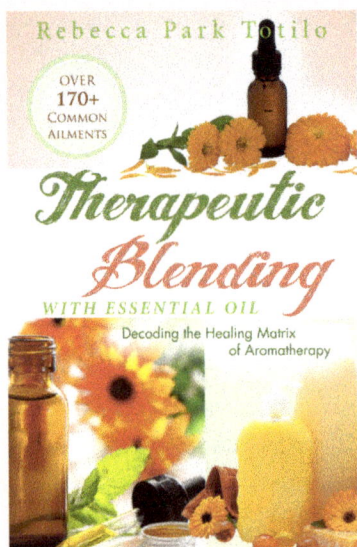

Therapeutic Blending With Essential Oil: Decoding the Healing Matrix of Aromatherapy

Therapeutic Blending With Essential Oil unlocks the healing power of essential oils and guides you through the intricate matrix of aromatherapy, with a compilation of over 170 common ailments. Discover how to properly formulate a blend for any physical or emotional symptom with easy to follow customizable recipes. Now, you can make your own massage oils, hand and body lotions, bath gels, compresses, salve ointments, smelling salts, nasal inhalers and more. This exhaustive guide takes all the guesswork out of blending oils from how many drops to include in a blend, to measuring thick oils, to how often to apply it for acute or chronic conditions. It also shows you how to create a single blend for multiple conditions. Even if you run out of oil for a favorite recipe, this book shows you how to substitute it with another oil.

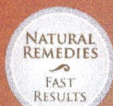

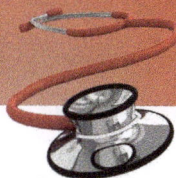

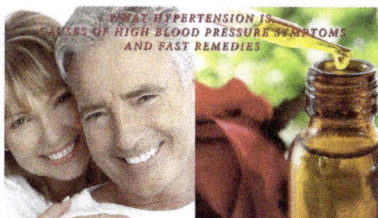

How To Lower Blood Pressure Naturally With Essential Oil: What Hypertension Is, Causes of High Pressure Symptoms and Fast Remedies

One out of three adults have it, and another one-third don't realize it. Oftentimes, it goes undetected for years. Even those who take multiple medications for it still don't have it under control. It's no secret—high blood pressure is rampant in America. High blood pressure, or hypertension, has become a household term. Between balancing meds and monitoring diets though, are the true causes—and best treatments—hidden in the shadows? In How to Lower Blood Pressure Naturally With Essential Oil, Rebecca Park Totilo sheds light on what high blood pressure is, the causes and symptoms of high blood pressure, and which essential oils regulate blood pressure and how to use essential oils as a natural, alternative method.

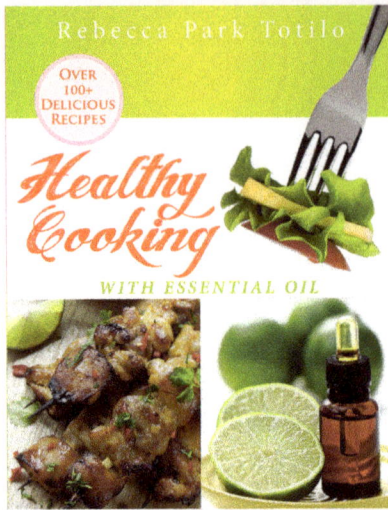

Healthy Cooking with Essential Oil

Imagine transforming an everyday dish into something extraordinary using only a drop or two of Essential oils can enliven everything from soups, salads, to main dishes and desserts. Boasting flavor and fragrance, these intense essences can turn a dull, boring meal into something appetizing and delicious. Essential oils are fun, easy-to use and beneficial, compared to the traditional stale, dried herbs and spices found in most pantries today. Healthy food should never be thought of as mere fuel for the body, it should be enjoyed as a multi-sensory experience that brings therapeutic value as well as nourishment. For years we have limited the use of essential oils to scented candles and soaps, in the belief that they were unsafe to consume (and some are!). However, more people are realizing the value of using pure essential oils to enhance their diet. In Healthy Cooking With Essential Oil, you will learn how cooking with essential oils can open up a wealth of creative opportunities in the kitchen.

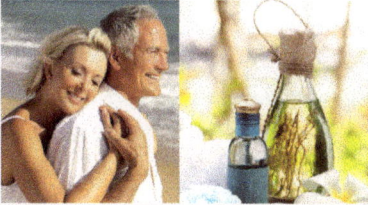

How to Lower Cholesterol with Essential Oil

Take healthy steps now to control high cholesterol and its risk factors with essential oils. People with high cholesterol have twice the risk for heart disease according to the Center for Disease Control and Prevention. What's worse, most folks aren't even aware that they have atherosclerosis until they have a heart attack or stroke. Lowering your cholesterol and triglycerides with essential oils may slow, reduce, or even stop the buildup of dangerous plaque in your arteries causing blockage of blood flow which could result in a heart attack or stroke. In this indispensable guide, author Rebecca Park Totilo presents scientific research supporting the efficacy of certain essential oils for lowering cholesterol, an extensive essential oil and carrier oil directory, natural treatments with recipes, along with easy-to-follow methods of use via inhalation, topically, and ingestion.

www.ingramcontent.com/pod-product-compliance
Lightning Source LLC
Chambersburg PA
CBHW051433270326
41935CB00018B/1816